AuDHD (Autism + ADHD) Complete Living Guide

Practical Strategies for Understanding, Managing, and Thriving

Gaetana Yo Tate

ISBN: 978-1-7641437-4-5

Isohan Publishing

Table of Contents

Chapter 1: The AuDHD Experience

More Than the Sum of Its Parts

AuDHD is a term you hear a lot these days, isn't it? It's shorthand for the experience of having both **autism** and **ADHD** (Attention-Deficit/Hyperactivity Disorder). While it's not an official diagnosis you'll find in a doctor's book, it describes a very real and often intense way of being in the world. Think of it as a widely accepted way to talk about something many people feel inside.

We know that autism and ADHD often show up together. Research shows a good number of people with autism also meet the criteria for ADHD, and vice versa. Before 2013, the diagnostic manual, the DSM-5, said you couldn't get both diagnoses. Imagine that! It was like saying you couldn't have both a head cold and a sprained ankle at the same time. This changed things in a big way. Allowing co-diagnosis was a game-changer because it finally gave people a way to explain their full experience.

The Weight of Missed Diagnoses

Think about what it must have been like before 2013, or even now, if you're an adult only just figuring things out. For so many years, countless individuals walked around with only half the story, or no story at all. Some got an **autism diagnosis** but their ADHD traits were missed, leading to struggles with things like **organization** or **impulsivity** that didn't quite fit the typical autism picture. Others received an **ADHD diagnosis** but their need for **routine, sensory sensitivities,** or **social communication differences** were overlooked, leaving them feeling baffled by their own reactions in social settings or overwhelmed by changes in plans.

Imagine a bright child, let's call her **Sarah**. From a young age, Sarah loved to line up her toys in perfect rows and knew everything there was to know about dinosaurs. But she also struggled to sit still in class, often blurted out answers, and lost her homework every other day. Her parents were told she had ADHD, and that explained her restlessness and distractibility. But no one really addressed her deep need for specific routines or her distress when the school fire alarm went off, which made her cling to her teacher for the rest of the day. As an adult, Sarah found herself constantly battling an internal conflict. She craved predictability, yet couldn't stick to a schedule to save her life. This internal tug-of-war left her feeling like a failure, always wondering why she couldn't just get it together. If only she had known about AuDHD earlier, she might have understood that these seemingly opposing traits were part of a single, understandable experience.

Or consider **Michael**, a quiet man who excelled at his computer programming job, often hyperfocusing for hours on complex code. But he struggled with deadlines, often starting projects at the last minute, and found team meetings excruciatingly draining. He'd been told he was "just shy" or "a bit quirky." It wasn't until his late 30s, after experiencing severe burnout, that he started researching his struggles. He discovered that his need for specific work environments (quiet, predictable), his intense focus on his interests, and his social anxieties pointed to autism, while his procrastination and difficulty with follow-through screamed ADHD. For years, he thought he was simply lazy or socially inept. Understanding AuDHD brought a wave of relief, helping him reframe his past and approach his present with new tools.

These past missteps in diagnosis, or the complete lack of it, didn't just leave people confused; they caused real harm. It led to **misguided therapies, self-blame**, and a deep sense of **not belonging**. When you don't have a name for what you're experiencing, it's hard to find others who feel the same, and it's even harder to ask for the right kind of help. The profound impact of these missed opportunities can last a lifetime, shaping self-perception and limiting potential.

The "Dual Operating System" Analogy

Now, let's talk about what makes AuDHD such a unique experience. Think of your brain as running two operating systems at once, and sometimes, they give conflicting commands. One system (the autistic side) craves **order, routine, predictability, and deep, specific interests**. The other system (the ADHD side) yearns for **novelty, spontaneity, excitement, and quick shifts in attention**. This isn't just theory; it plays out in everyday life in ways that can be both bewildering and frustrating.

Take **routine**, for example. Someone with AuDHD might deeply desire a set routine for their morning, down to the exact order of putting on their socks. This gives them comfort and a sense of control. Yet, their ADHD brain might rebel against that very routine, making it incredibly hard to initiate tasks, leading to frequent diversions, or suddenly feeling an urge to do something completely different. This can lead to a constant internal battle, leaving you exhausted before the day even begins.

Consider **planning a trip**. The autistic side might want every detail meticulously planned: reservations, exact timings, knowing exactly what to expect. The ADHD side might find this level of detail overwhelming and boring, leading to procrastination in planning, a desire to spontaneously change plans, or leaving things to the last minute, which then clashes with the need for predictability. Imagine wanting to travel but hating the idea of travel because it disrupts your routine, yet also getting bored easily and craving the excitement of a new place. It's a real paradox.

Then there's **hyperfocus**. This amazing ability to concentrate intensely on one thing. For an autistic person, this might mean spending hours researching a specific topic, like the migratory patterns of a rare bird, to the exclusion of everything else. For someone with ADHD, hyperfocus might appear when they're suddenly captivated by a new project or idea, becoming completely absorbed until the novelty wears off. With AuDHD, you might get both. You might **hyperfocus** on your **special interest**, only to find yourself getting distracted by a new, shiny object just as easily. Or, you might find your **hyperfocus** is directed towards something totally unplanned, making it hard to shift to what you "should" be doing.

Example 1: The Kitchen Chaos

Liam, who has AuDHD, knows he functions best when his kitchen is tidy and organized. He has a precise way of arranging his spices and dishes, which brings him a lot of comfort (autistic trait). However, when he cooks, his ADHD kicks in. He starts several cooking tasks at once, gets distracted by a podcast, forgets to put ingredients away immediately, and suddenly the kitchen is a disaster zone.

The sight of the mess then causes him immense distress because it violates his need for order. This cycle of wanting order but struggling to maintain it due to executive function challenges is a classic AuDHD clash. He'll then spend hours fixing the kitchen, sometimes hyperfocusing on the cleaning process, only to repeat the cycle days later.

Example 2: Social Gatherings and Internal Battles

Chloe looks forward to her friend's birthday party, knowing exactly what she wants to wear and what time she needs to leave. She even mentally rehearses a few conversation starters (autistic planning). But as the time approaches, her ADHD brain starts craving something new. She suddenly feels an intense urge to stay home and finish a new craft project she just started, or perhaps go to a different, spontaneous event her other friend just mentioned. She pushes through to go to the party, but once there, her need for quiet conversation clashes with the loud music and shifting groups of people (sensory sensitivity, social difference). She finds herself struggling to follow multiple conversations, getting easily overstimulated, and then feels a strong pull to escape the overwhelming environment, perhaps by retreating to a quiet corner and hyperfocusing on her phone.

This "dual operating system" means your brain can feel like a perpetual debate club. It's not that you're being difficult or uncooperative; it's that two powerful, often contradictory, forces are at play inside you. This makes simple tasks feel complicated and daily life a constant navigation challenge.

This chapter starts by saying, "This book is for you who may feel **'too much'** or **'not enough'**." That phrase hits home for many AuDHD individuals. You might feel "too much" because your intensity, your sensory reactions, or your sudden bursts of energy can overwhelm others. Or you might feel "not enough" because you struggle with basic organization, remembering appointments, or keeping up with neurotypical social cues, leaving you feeling inadequate in a world not built for your brain. This book aims to show you that these feelings are valid, that your experience is real, and that you are not alone. It's about recognizing the uniqueness of your internal world and giving you tools to navigate it with confidence.

Key Takeaways

- AuDHD describes the common experience of having both autism and ADHD, a co-occurrence now recognized by the DSM-5 since 2013.

- Past missed diagnoses caused significant self-blame and misunderstanding, highlighting the need for a complete picture of one's neurology.

- The AuDHD brain often operates like a "dual system," where the autistic need for routine and special interests can clash with the ADHD desire for novelty and spontaneous attention shifts.

- Hyperfocus can arise from both autistic intensity and ADHD novelty-seeking, leading to powerful, sometimes hard-to-direct, concentration.

- Feeling "too much" or "not enough" is a common AuDHD experience, and this book validates those feelings while offering practical guidance.

Chapter 2: Unmasking Your Authentic Self

It's easy to get caught up in the challenges of AuDHD, isn't it? The missed appointments, the sensory overload, the social missteps. But what if we flipped the script? What if we looked at these very traits, sometimes seen as deficits, as sources of **incredible strength**? That's what this chapter is all about. It's about recognizing the unique advantages your AuDHD brain brings to the table – your **superpowers**, if you will.

Your brain works differently, yes, and that difference often translates into extraordinary abilities. Think about it:

- **Inventive problem-solving:** Because you see the world from a different angle, you often come up with solutions others never would. You're not tied to conventional thinking. Imagine a puzzle where everyone is trying to fit square pegs into square holes, but you—because your brain works differently—see that some pegs are actually triangles and there are triangle holes hidden in plain sight.

  - **Case Example: The Disorganized Office.** *Maria* worked in an office where files were constantly misplaced, and everyone complained about the inefficient system. Her colleagues tried to reorganize folders by color or alphabetically, but nothing stuck. Maria, with her AuDHD brain, noticed not only the lack of organization (an ADHD struggle she knew well) but also the sensory overload from the cluttered desks (an autistic sensitivity).

7

She proposed a system that wasn't just about labeling, but about creating **visual cues** for each project type, assigning **specific, distinct areas** for different tasks, and using **noise-canceling headphones** during periods of intense focus. She even designed a "return to sender" box for items that didn't have a clear home. Her boss, at first skeptical, found that Maria's system, though unconventional, dramatically reduced misfiles and improved workflow, all because she addressed both the executive function and sensory aspects of the problem. Her ability to **hyperfocus** on systematizing and her **keen observation** of the environmental stressors allowed her to create an inventive, personalized solution.

- **Deep curiosity:** When something truly grabs your interest, you go all in. This isn't just a casual interest; it's a **quest for knowledge,** a desire to know everything there is to know about a topic. This can lead to expertise in unexpected areas.

- **Strong moral compass:** Many AuDHD individuals have a powerful sense of justice and fairness. You feel things deeply, and if something isn't right, you often feel a strong urge to speak up. This can make you a powerful advocate for others.

- **Keen observation:** You notice details others miss. Whether it's a slight change in someone's tone of voice, a pattern in data, or a small inconsistency in an argument, your ability to pick up on these nuances can be a true asset.

- **Resilience:** You've probably faced a lot of challenges and misunderstandings. Each time you've picked yourself up, you've built a stronger inner core. You've adapted, often creatively, to a world that sometimes doesn't quite get you.

- **Humor:** There's a particular kind of wit often found in neurodivergent brains—a dry, unexpected, or incredibly clever sense of humor that can lighten any situation.

- **Originality:** You don't necessarily follow the crowd. Your thoughts, ideas, and ways of expressing yourself are genuinely your own, leading to truly innovative contributions.

- **Hyperfocus when aligned with interests:** We talked about hyperfocus as a "dual operating system" challenge, but when it aligns with something you love or a task that needs doing, it becomes an incredible asset. You can achieve in hours what might take others days, simply because you can shut out distractions and drill down.

  - **Case Example: The Coding Prodigy.** *David,* an AuDHD software developer, found conventional work environments stifling. He struggled with small talk, couldn't stand the fluorescent lights, and constantly felt overwhelmed by office chatter. However, when given a complex coding challenge that interested him, he could disappear into it for 12 hours straight, forgetting to eat or sleep. His **autistic drive** for systems and logical precision combined with his **ADHD capacity**

for intense, sustained attention (when interested) made him uniquely capable of solving highly technical, difficult problems that stumped his neurotypical peers. He wasn't just good; he was exceptionally good, able to see patterns and write elegant code because he could immerse himself completely in the logic.

The Weight of Masking

Now, let's get real about something many AuDHD individuals do without even realizing it: **masking**. Think of masking as putting on a performance, a social costume, to fit in. You learn what's expected in different situations and try your best to act "normal." This might mean forcing yourself to make eye contact even when it feels uncomfortable, suppressing your stims (repetitive movements like fidgeting or rocking), or scripting conversations so you know what to say. For people with ADHD, masking might involve trying desperately to appear organized and attentive when your mind is actually buzzing. For autistic people, it might be about trying to mimic social cues or feign interest in small talk.

The problem? Masking is exhausting. It takes an incredible amount of mental energy to constantly monitor your behavior, suppress your natural reactions, and pretend to be someone you're not. This constant performance wears you down, leading to **burnout, anxiety**, and even **depression**. It also creates a barrier between your authentic self and the world, making it hard for others to truly know and accept you. When you're masking, you're essentially telling yourself that who you truly are isn't good enough, which can chip away at your **self-esteem** and **identity**.

Imagine *Alex*, a young adult with AuDHD. In social settings, Alex would force himself to maintain constant eye contact, even though it felt painful. He'd practice jokes he heard on TV to use in conversation and try to seem interested in topics he found boring. After every social event, Alex would feel utterly drained, often needing days to recover. This constant effort led to a deep sense of loneliness, because even surrounded by people, he felt nobody truly saw *him*. His masking also hid his true needs, like preferring quiet spaces or needing clear, direct communication, which meant he rarely got the accommodations that would make his life easier.

Beginning Your Unmasking Journey

The idea of unmasking can feel scary, like shedding armor you've worn your whole life. But it's also incredibly freeing. It's about slowly, gently, letting your authentic self show. This isn't about throwing caution to the wind and abandoning all social graces. It's about being more of *you* in situations where it feels safe and right.

Here are some gentle steps to begin this journey:

1. **Self-Observation Without Judgment:** Start by simply noticing. What do you do naturally when you're alone and comfortable? Do you fidget? Pace? Hum? What feels good to you? Do this without telling yourself it's "wrong" or "weird." It's just you being you. This builds **self-awareness**.

2. **Identify Your "Masking Triggers":** What situations make you feel the need to mask the most? Is it job interviews? Family gatherings? Certain types of social

events? Knowing your triggers helps you prepare or choose to limit exposure.

3. **Find Safe Spaces and Safe People:** Begin by unmasking in environments where you feel genuinely accepted. This might be with a close friend, a family member who understands, a therapist, or a neurodiversity support group. Practice being more yourself with people who already care about you.

    o **Case Example: The Comfort of True Friends.** *Jamal* always felt the need to present a highly organized, calm exterior at work, despite his internal chaos. He'd spend hours before meetings preparing, trying to anticipate every question, and making sure he sounded articulate. But with his two closest friends, he slowly started to unmask. He admitted his struggles with executive function, letting them see his messy apartment, and openly stimmed by quietly rocking when he was anxious. His friends, rather than judging, offered practical help and genuine understanding. This experience of **acceptance** helped Jamal realize that being himself didn't mean losing friendships; it meant building deeper, more authentic ones.

4. **Experiment with Small Unmasking Actions:** You don't have to overhaul your entire personality overnight. Try one small thing. Maybe it's allowing yourself to fidget with a small object during a casual conversation. Or using your natural tone of voice

instead of a practiced one. Or asking a clarifying question instead of pretending to understand.

5. **Communicate Your Needs (When Appropriate):** Instead of forcing yourself to conform, try politely explaining your needs. "I process information better if I can write it down," or "I sometimes need quiet to concentrate." This isn't about making excuses; it's about setting yourself up for success.

6. **Celebrate Your Neurodivergent Traits:** Start to see your AuDHD as a part of what makes you uniquely capable. Your **hyperfocus** can make you a master of your chosen field. Your **attention to detail** can make you a fantastic editor or artist. Your **original thinking** can make you an innovator. This reframing is a powerful step towards self-acceptance.

Unmasking is a process, not a destination. It's about **self-acceptance** and building a life where you feel more at ease being you. This chapter aims to kickstart that process, setting a **neurodiversity-affirming tone** for the whole book. You are enough, just as you are. And discovering your authentic self is one of the most freeing things you'll ever do.

Key Takeaways

- Common AuDHD traits like unique problem-solving, deep curiosity, a strong moral compass, sharp observation, resilience, humor, originality, and hyperfocus are powerful strengths.

- **Masking** (camouflaging neurodivergent traits) drains mental energy, leads to burnout, and hurts **self-esteem**.

- Unmasking is a gradual process of allowing your authentic self to show in safe environments.

- Steps to unmasking involve self-observation, identifying triggers, finding safe spaces, small experiments, communicating needs, and celebrating your neurodivergent traits.

When we talk about living with AuDHD, it isn't about fixing something that's broken. It's about recognizing the incredible way your brain works and learning to work *with* it, not against it. Think of it as learning the instruction manual for a truly remarkable, bespoke piece of machinery. You've got strengths that many would envy, and with the right understanding, you can bring those strengths to the world in ways that feel good to you. Keep this thought close: you are not a problem to be solved; you are a complex, brilliant individual ready to thrive.

Chapter 3: Mastering Executive Function

Dealing with executive function challenges can feel like trying to herd cats while juggling—it's chaotic, messy, and things often drop. For someone with AuDHD, these challenges are often magnified, creating a perfect storm of difficulty with everyday tasks. We're talking about things like starting a project, keeping track of steps, organizing our stuff, knowing how much time something will take, and holding information in our minds just long enough to use it. These aren't character flaws; they are simply how our brains process and organize the world. The good news is, we can build bridges over these choppy waters.

Understanding the AuDHD Executive Function Blend

Let's break down some common executive function hurdles. **Task initiation** can be a big one—that feeling of being stuck at the starting line, even when you know what to do. It's not laziness; it's a disconnect between knowing and doing. **Planning and organization** often go hand-in-hand, making it tough to map out steps or keep our physical and digital spaces tidy. Think of the paperwork piles that seem to multiply on their own, or the forgotten appointments that pop up like unwelcome surprises.

Then there's **time blindness**, a common experience where time feels more like a suggestion than a strict rule. Five minutes can feel like an hour, and an hour can vanish in a blink. This makes planning difficult and showing up on time a consistent struggle. Finally, **working memory deficits** mean holding information in your mind while you're using it can be a true test. You might forget what you walked into a room for, or lose your train of thought mid-sentence. For AuDHDers, these aspects combine; the ADHD part might make you forget where you put something in a burst of activity, while the autistic need for order gets frustrated by the mess. It's a tricky balance, but one we can certainly navigate.

Tools for Tackling Executive Function Challenges

We don't need to reinvent the wheel here; we simply need the right tools in our toolbox. Many tried-and-true methods shine particularly bright for the AuDHD mind.

Visual schedules are a true friend. For someone who struggles with time blindness or remembering multi-step processes, seeing the day laid out can be a game-changer. This can be as simple as a whiteboard with "Wake Up," "Eat Breakfast," "Get Dressed," and so on, using pictures or words. For a more detailed day, you could use a digital calendar with color-coded blocks for different activities.

- **Case in Point: Sarah's Morning Routine** Sarah, a 32-year-old with AuDHD, used to face utter chaos every morning. She would often forget steps, get distracted, and end up running late for work, feeling stressed before her day even began. We worked together to create a visual schedule. She used a large corkboard in her kitchen and printed out cards with icons and short descriptions: a picture of a toothbrush for "Brush Teeth," a bowl of cereal for "Eat Breakfast," and a shirt for "Get Dressed." Each morning, she'd move the card from a "To Do" pocket to a "Done" pocket. This simple visual cue helped her stay on track, reduced her anxiety about forgetting something, and gave her a sense of accomplishment as she moved each card. She told me, "It's like my brain finally has a map instead of just a compass spinning wildly."

Checklists are another amazing ally. Whether it's a grocery list, a packing list, or a list for a work project, checking things off provides a clear path and a satisfying sense of progress. For people who feel overwhelmed by the sheer volume of things to do, breaking tasks down into smaller, tickable items lessens the load considerably.

Timers are a secret weapon against time blindness. Setting a timer for specific tasks can help you focus, provide a clear end point, and prevent you from losing track of how much time has passed. The Pomodoro Technique—working for 25 minutes, then taking a 5-minute break—works well for many with AuDHD, offering structured focus periods that respect attention span fluctuations.

- **Case in Point: Alex's Project Deadline** Alex, a graphic designer, found starting and completing large design projects extremely difficult. He'd often get stuck in research for hours, losing track of time, or feel overwhelmed by the project's scale. We introduced him to using a visual timer. For his next project, he broke it down: "Concept Sketching (30 minutes)," "Color Palette Selection (20 minutes)," "Initial Digital Draft (45 minutes)." He set a bright, physical timer for each block. When the timer went off, he knew it was time to switch tasks, even if he wasn't "finished." This method helped him move through the project more efficiently, preventing him from getting stuck in one phase for too long, and helped him recognize how long tasks actually took.

Calendar applications are practically magic for managing appointments and deadlines. Digital calendars with reminders are perfect because they can send you notifications across your devices, acting as a gentle nudge when your brain might otherwise forget. Color-coding events can help, too, making it easy to see different categories of commitments at a glance.

Breaking Down Big Tasks

The idea of "eating the elephant one bite at a time" is particularly apt here. Large tasks often feel like an insurmountable mountain. But by breaking them into **manageable "chunks,"** that mountain becomes a series of smaller, more achievable hills.

1. **Identify the end goal:** What does "done" look like?

2. **Brainstorm all steps:** Write down every single thing you can think of that needs to happen to get to the end goal, no matter how small.

3. **Order the steps:** Put them in a logical sequence.

4. **Group small steps:** Combine related small steps into slightly larger, more manageable chunks.

5. **Assign realistic timeframes:** How long will each chunk truly take? Be honest with yourself.

6. **Schedule chunks:** Put these chunks into your calendar or visual schedule.

- **Case in Point: Maria's Apartment Declutter** Maria felt constantly overwhelmed by the clutter in her apartment. The idea of "decluttering the whole apartment" was so huge it paralyzed her. We reframed it. The goal was a calmer living space.

- **Instead of:** "Clean the apartment."
- **We broke it down into:**
  - "Declutter kitchen counter (15 minutes)"
  - "Sort mail (10 minutes)"
  - "Put away clothes in bedroom (20 minutes)"
  - "Organize one shelf in the living room (30 minutes)" By focusing on these small, specific tasks, Maria started making progress. She could choose one "chunk" each day, and slowly, the mountain began to shrink, replaced by noticeable improvements.

Creating Designated "Homes" and Managing Paper Clutter

Disorganization is a thief of time and peace of mind. For people with AuDHD, the sensory overload of clutter combined with the difficulty of remembering where things go can be a perfect recipe for chaos. The solution? **Give everything a "home."**

Think of your items like pets—they need their own specific spot. When you're done with something, it goes back to its home. This isn't about rigid perfection; it's about reducing mental load. If your keys always go on the hook by the door, you don't have to waste precious working memory searching for them every morning.

- **For physical items:**
  - **Hooks by the door** for keys, bags, coats.
  - **Labeled bins or drawers** for specific categories (e.g., "batteries," "craft supplies," "electronic chargers").
  - **Clear containers** so you can see what's inside without having to open them all.
  - **A "landing strip"** near the entrance for incoming mail, bags, and shoes.

- **For paper clutter:** Oh, the paper! It arrives, it multiplies, it forms menacing stacks.
  - **The "One Touch" Rule:** Try to handle paper only once. When mail comes in, immediately sort it into: **Shred, File, Action,** or **Recycle.**
  - **A dedicated inbox:** Have one specific tray or basket for incoming paper that needs attention. Don't let it spread across surfaces.
  - **Simple filing system:** A basic accordion file with categories like "Bills to Pay," "Important Documents," "Medical," and "Receipts" can work wonders. Avoid overly complex systems you won't keep up with.
  - **Go digital where possible:** Sign up for e-statements, pay bills online, and scan important documents. Reduce the amount of paper entering your home.

- Case in Point: David's Desk Dilemma

David's home office desk was a battleground of papers, half-finished projects, and random gadgets. This made it hard for him to focus, and he often lost important documents. We tackled it by creating "homes."

- He installed a **key hook** right by his office door.

- He got a simple **three-tier inbox** for his desk: "To Sort," "To Action," and "To File."

- For cables and small electronics, he used a **drawer organizer** with labeled compartments.

- Crucially, he made it a habit to **process his "To Sort" inbox for 10 minutes** at the end of each workday. It wasn't about clearing everything, but making steady progress. He found this routine surprisingly calming and effective.

Flexible Routines for Reduced Overwhelm

The AuDHD brain loves routine but can also rebel against rigidity. The key is **flexible routines**. This means having a general structure but allowing for natural variations. Think of it less like a military drill and more like a gentle river—it has a course, but it can flow around obstacles.

- **Daily "anchors":** Identify 2-3 non-negotiable activities that happen at roughly the same time each day, like a morning routine, a lunchtime break, or an evening wind-down. These act as touchstones.

- **Time blocking, not time dictating:** Instead of saying "I will work on X from 9:00 AM to 10:00 AM," say "I will work on X during my morning 'focus block,' whenever that starts." This reduces the pressure if you're running a bit behind.

- **"If-Then" planning:** "If I finish my work task, then I will take a 10-minute walk." This helps with transitions and motivation.

- **Build in "transition time":** AuDHD brains often need extra time to switch gears. Schedule 5-10 minutes between tasks to decompress, stretch, or do something calming.

- **Account for "AuDHD Tax":** Add extra time to every estimate for potential distractions, sensory issues, or task switching difficulties. If you think something will take 30 minutes, schedule 45. This builds in grace and reduces last-minute panic.

- Case in Point: Maya's Evening Struggle

Maya, a college student, found her evenings spiraling into last-minute cramming and skipped meals because she couldn't transition from classes to studying to self-care. We created a flexible evening routine:

- **Anchor:** Dinner between 6 PM and 7 PM.

- **After class:** "Decompression time" (30 minutes of listening to music or reading for pleasure).

- **Study block:** 2 hours, broken into 45-minute Pomodoros.

- **Evening wind-down:** 30 minutes of screen-free time before bed. If a class ran late, she wouldn't panic; she'd just shift the start of her decompression time. The flexibility reduced her stress significantly.

By understanding how executive functions work for AuDHD and equipping ourselves with these practical tools, we can move from a state of constant overwhelm to purposeful action. It's about designing a system that works *with* our brains, not against them.

Key Takeaways

- AuDHD often presents challenges with task initiation, planning, organization, time perception, and working memory. These are not character flaws but differences in brain processing.

- Tools like **visual schedules, checklists, timers, and calendar applications** provide external structure and support that our brains find helpful.

- Breaking down large tasks into **smaller, manageable "chunks"** makes them less daunting and more achievable.

- Giving every item a **designated "home"** and using simple systems for paper clutter drastically reduces mental load and visual chaos.

- **Flexible routines** with daily anchors, transition time, and an "AuDHD Tax" allow for structure without rigidity, reducing overwhelm and supporting natural variations in our energy and focus.

Chapter 4: Sensory Sanctuary

Creating Your Ideal Environment

Imagine living in a world where every sound is amplified, every light is glaring, every texture is irritating, and every scent is overpowering. For many with AuDHD, this is not an exaggeration; it's daily life. The compounded sensory sensitivities are a major pain point, leading to quick burnout, anxiety, and a feeling of being constantly on edge. When your sensory system is constantly on high alert, simply existing can feel exhausting. But here's the hopeful part: we can actively shape our environments to be sanctuaries, places that nurture rather than deplete us.

Understanding Compounded Sensory Sensitivities

People with autism often experience sensory input more intensely than neurotypical individuals—a phenomenon known as **sensory hyper-sensitivity**. Simultaneously, individuals with ADHD can have difficulty filtering out irrelevant stimuli, meaning their brains are trying to process *everything* at once. Put these two together, and you have a sensory system that is both highly sensitive *and* easily overwhelmed. A faint hum might be painfully loud, or the texture of a shirt could be unbearable. Bright lights can cause headaches, and strong smells might lead to nausea. The constant bombardment of sensory information drains energy and makes it incredibly difficult to focus, regulate emotions, or simply feel at ease. This isn't just about discomfort; it directly impacts our ability to function, learn, and connect with the world around us.

Actionable Strategies for Managing Sensory Overload

The first step to creating a sanctuary is to reduce the input that causes distress. This often means actively blocking or modifying sensory experiences.

- **Noise-Canceling Headphones:** These are often considered a lifeline. Whether it's the hum of an office, the chatter in a coffee shop, or just the general sounds of home, good noise-canceling headphones can create a pocket of quiet. They can be used for short breaks, during focus tasks, or even just to buffer the world when you're feeling overwhelmed. Some people prefer active noise-canceling, which uses technology to cancel out sound waves, while others find passive noise-isolating headphones (which physically block sound) more comfortable. Experiment to find what works best for you.

- **Tinted Glasses or Blue Light Filters:** Fluorescent lights, bright screens, and even natural daylight can be too intense. **Tinted glasses** (amber, rose, or even slightly gray) can significantly reduce visual overload without making everything too dark. **Blue light filtering glasses** or screen settings can also help, especially for those sensitive to the harsh blue light emitted by devices, which can contribute to eye strain and disrupt sleep.

- **Dim Lighting:** Bright, overhead lighting is often a culprit for sensory distress. Opt for **dimmable lights, lamps with warmer bulbs**, or even **fairy lights** to create a softer, more inviting glow. Natural light, when not too intense, is often preferred, but sometimes even that needs to be softened with sheer curtains or blinds.

- **Establishing Quiet Spaces:** This is about having a designated spot—even a small one—where you can retreat and recover. This doesn't have to be an entire room. It could be a cozy corner with a comfortable chair, a bedroom that's free of distractions, or even just a specific spot under a desk. The goal is a place where you can reduce sensory input and allow your nervous system to calm down. Communicate to others in your household that this space is for quiet and calm, so they understand when you need to use it.

- Case in Point: Jessica's Overwhelming Commute

Jessica's commute on public transport left her drained before her workday even began. The cacophony of voices, train announcements, and street noise was unbearable. She started using high-quality noise-canceling headphones and playing gentle, instrumental music or white noise. She also switched to wearing tinted sunglasses even on cloudy days to soften the visual input from windows and advertising. This simple addition made her commute tolerable, and she arrived at work feeling far less agitated. She said it was like "a bubble of peace" in the middle of the noise.

Incorporating Sensory-Seeking Behaviors for Self-Regulation

It's not just about reducing negative input; it's also about providing positive, regulating sensory experiences. Sensory-seeking behaviors, often called **stimming** (short for self-stimulatory behavior), are crucial for self-regulation in AuDHD individuals. These actions help our nervous systems process information, manage stress, and release excess energy. They are not something to suppress, but rather to understand and incorporate constructively.

- **Stimming:** This can take many forms: rocking, hand flapping, twirling hair, humming, repetitive movements, or even chewing. The key is that it helps you regulate. Recognize what stims help you and allow yourself to engage in them in safe and acceptable ways. Sometimes, redirecting a less socially accepted stim to a more discreet one (like using a fidget toy instead of hand flapping vigorously in a meeting) can be helpful.

- **Fidget Tools:** These are a fantastic way to provide sensory input and allow for discreet stimming. They come in endless varieties: spinner rings, textured stones, squishy balls, tangle toys, chewable jewelry, and more. Having a few different options available can be useful, as different textures or movements might be needed depending on your current sensory needs.

- **Weighted Blankets:** The gentle, even pressure of a **weighted blanket** can be incredibly calming and grounding. It provides deep pressure input, which many people with AuDHD find soothing for anxiety, sensory overload, and sleep difficulties. It's like a comforting hug for your nervous system. These blankets are typically 10-15% of your body weight.

- Case in Point: Liam's Classroom Focus

Liam, a high school student, struggled to focus in class, often tapping his pencil or fidgeting restlessly. His teachers saw it as disruptive. After understanding his AuDHD, his parents provided him with a fidget cube and a chewable necklace. He also started using a small weighted lap pad during longer lectures. These tools allowed him to quietly channel his need for movement and sensory input, helping him pay attention and process information without disturbing others. His grades improved, and his teachers reported a noticeable decrease in disruptive behaviors.

Designing Sensory-Friendly Home and Personal Environments

Creating a sensory sanctuary is an ongoing process of observation, experimentation, and adjustment. It's about tailoring your surroundings to your unique sensory profile.

- **Lighting Control:** As discussed, prioritize dimmable lights, warmer LED bulbs (2700K-3000K), and indirect lighting. Consider smart bulbs that allow you to adjust color temperature and brightness. Use natural light where possible, but have blinds or curtains ready to diffuse it if it's too bright.

- **Soundscapes:** Beyond noise-canceling headphones, consider what sounds are calming. For some, it's complete silence. For others, it's white noise, nature sounds (rain, ocean waves), or soft instrumental music. Explore sound machines or apps that offer these options. Acoustic panels or thick rugs can also help absorb sound in a room.

- **Texture and Fabric Choices:** Pay attention to how different materials feel against your skin. Opt for soft, natural fibers for clothing, bedding, and upholstery. Avoid scratchy tags—cut them out! If certain textures are particularly soothing, incorporate them into your environment, like a soft throw blanket or a plush rug.

- **Minimalism and Organization:** Clutter creates visual noise, which can be overwhelming. A more minimalist approach, with less visual distraction, can contribute to a calmer environment. This ties back to the executive function chapter: designated "homes" for items reduce visual chaos and make spaces feel more orderly.

- **Scent Management:** Strong scents—perfumes, cleaning products, air fresheners—can be highly irritating. Opt for unscented products whenever possible. If you like scents, use natural essential oils sparingly and choose calming aromas like lavender or chamomile, diffusing them gently rather than using strong sprays. Ensure good ventilation to air out any offending smells quickly.

- **Temperature Control:** Being too hot or too cold can be a significant sensory irritant. Ensure you have comfortable temperature control in your living and working spaces. Layers of clothing can help you adjust throughout the day.

- Case in Point: Sarah's Living Room Oasis

Remember Sarah from Chapter 3? Her living room used to be a source of stress due to harsh lighting and overwhelming clutter. We transformed it into a sensory oasis.

  - She replaced her bright overhead light with a **dimmable floor lamp** and added a few smaller lamps with warm-toned bulbs.

- She put up **thick, blackout curtains** to control natural light and muffle outside noise.

- She invested in a **super-soft, weighted blanket** for her couch and a couple of plush throw pillows.

- She created a "fidget basket" with various **fidget toys** and stress balls, easily accessible.

- She cleared out excess decor, creating a more **minimalist space** that felt less visually busy. Sarah now finds her living room to be a genuine sanctuary, a place where she can unwind and regulate after a long day, rather than feeling constantly overwhelmed by her surroundings.

Creating a sensory sanctuary is not about escaping the world, but about making it more manageable. By mindfully adjusting our environments and incorporating tools that support our unique sensory needs, we can significantly reduce daily discomfort and create spaces where we feel safe, calm, and truly at home.

Key Takeaways

- AuDHD often leads to compounded sensory sensitivities, making everyday environments overwhelming and draining.

- Strategies to manage sensory overload include using **noise-canceling headphones, tinted glasses, dim lighting, and establishing quiet spaces** for retreat.

- **Sensory-seeking behaviors like stimming and using fidget tools** are vital for self-regulation and should be acknowledged and supported.

- **Weighted blankets** provide deep pressure input that can be incredibly calming for anxiety and sensory overload.

- Designing sensory-friendly environments involves paying attention to **lighting, soundscapes, textures, organization, scents, and temperature control** to create spaces that nurture rather than deplete.

Chapter 5: Communication & Connection

Bridging the Neurotype Gap

When someone faces both ADHD and autism, the way they experience the world—and how they share that experience with others—is often something quite special. It's like having two unique filters through which all information passes, creating a way of processing that's truly one-of-a-kind. Sometimes, this can lead to wonderful new ideas and perspectives. Other times, it can make typical interactions feel a bit like trying to read a map upside down in the dark. But with a bit of clarity and a willingness to understand, those tricky spots can become opportunities for incredible connection.

Have you ever felt like you and another person were speaking completely different languages, even though you were using the same words? For many AuDHD individuals, this feeling is a common thread running through their daily conversations. It's not about being bad at communicating; it's about having a communication style that often doesn't quite line up with what neurotypical folks expect. This can show up in many ways—perhaps a struggle with the give-and-take of a conversation, a challenge picking up on subtle social clues, or even misunderstanding the true meaning behind someone's tone of voice or body language.

Think about it: a typical conversation is a bit like a dance. People take turns, respond to unspoken signals, and adjust their movements based on what the other person is doing. But if you're AuDHD, you might miss a beat or two, step on a toe, or just be doing a completely different dance altogether!

This isn't a deficit on your part; it's just a different rhythm. Understanding these differences is the first step toward creating spaces where everyone can communicate with less friction and more genuine connection.

How Communication Often Looks Different

For those with AuDHD, communication can be a fascinating study in contrasts. You might find yourself saying exactly what you mean, literally, only to discover that others expected you to read between the lines. This is a common point of confusion.

Consider **conversational flow**. Many neurotypical conversations involve quick back-and-forth exchanges, interruptions that are seen as enthusiastic participation, and a lot of implied understanding. For someone AuDHD, this can feel like a chaotic tennis match where the ball keeps changing direction without warning. You might need a moment to process what's been said before you can formulate a response, and by then, the conversation might have moved on. This can lead to feeling left out or constantly playing catch-up.

Then there are **social cues**. These are the silent signals—a raised eyebrow, a slight shift in posture, a quick glance—that convey so much in typical social interactions. For many AuDHD individuals, these cues can be incredibly difficult to interpret. It's like trying to decode a secret language without a key. Someone might be bored, annoyed, or excited, and you might not pick up on it, leading to misunderstandings or unintentional social missteps.

Understanding tone and body language also presents its own set of hurdles. Sarcasm, for instance, can be a real tripwire. A neurotypical person might use a playful tone to indicate they're joking, but an AuDHD person might take the words at face value. The same goes for body language. Crossed arms might mean someone is cold, while to others it signals defensiveness. These subtle variations can create a communication chasm, leading to frustration on both sides.

Let's look at an example. Sarah, an AuDHD individual, was at a team meeting. Her boss, Mr. Henderson, said, "Sarah, could you maybe look into that report by end of day?" Mr. Henderson thought his slightly stressed tone and the way he tapped his pen would convey urgency. Sarah, however, heard "maybe look into," interpreted it as low priority, and planned to get to it the next day after finishing her other tasks. The next morning, Mr. Henderson was frustrated that the report wasn't ready, and Sarah was confused, believing she had followed instructions. This is a classic case where implied meaning (urgency through tone and body language) was missed because Sarah processes language more literally.

Building Bridges: Strategies for Clear Communication

The good news is that we can build bridges across this communication gap. It begins with both sides making a conscious effort to adjust their approaches. For neurotypical individuals communicating with someone AuDHD, a key strategy is to **avoid subtext**. Say what you mean, directly and plainly. Don't rely on hints, sarcasm, or unspoken expectations. If you need something done by a certain time, state that time explicitly. If you're upset, say "I'm feeling upset," rather than expecting the other person to pick up on your sighing or slumped shoulders.

Offering **explicit explanations** is another game-changer. When giving instructions, break them down into clear, sequential steps. Don't assume anything is obvious. If you're talking about a concept, spell it out fully. This isn't about "dumbing down" information; it's about ensuring clarity and reducing ambiguity, which is a gift to anyone who processes information differently.

Think about a common scenario: a couple planning their weekend. Mark (AuDHD) asks his partner, Lisa, "What do you want to do this weekend?" Lisa replies, "Oh, whatever, I'm flexible." To Lisa, this means she's open to suggestions and wants Mark to take the lead. To Mark, "whatever" means she genuinely has no preference, and he might struggle to come up with ideas or worry he'll pick something she secretly dislikes. A better response from Lisa might be, "I'm open to ideas, but I'm feeling a bit tired, so maybe something low-key. What are you thinking?" This provides concrete information and a starting point.

Utilizing written communication can also be incredibly helpful, especially for clarifying tasks and responsibilities. Emails, texts, or shared digital documents can serve as clear, unambiguous records. This is particularly useful in professional settings or when discussing important household duties. A written list of chores, for instance, leaves less room for misinterpretation than a verbal discussion. It allows the AuDHD individual to refer back to the exact words, reducing anxiety about forgetting something or doing it incorrectly.

For instance, Maria, who has AuDHD, often found herself forgetting specific details of tasks assigned verbally at work. Her manager, recognizing this, started sending follow-up emails after every meeting summarizing action items, deadlines, and who was responsible for what. Maria found this incredibly helpful. She could refer to the email, check things off as she went, and feel much more confident that she was meeting expectations. This simple shift in communication style reduced her stress and increased her productivity.

The Double Empathy Problem: A Shift in Perspective

Here's a concept that can truly change how you see communication differences: **The Double Empathy Problem** [1]. For a long time, the prevailing idea was that autistic (and by extension, AuDHD) individuals lacked empathy or struggled to understand neurotypical social rules. This put the "problem" squarely on the neurodivergent person, suggesting they needed to be "fixed" to communicate effectively.

The Double Empathy Problem flips this on its head. It suggests that communication breakdowns between neurotypical and neurodivergent people are not solely due to a "deficit" in the neurodivergent individual. Instead, it posits that there's a **mutual lack of understanding**. Neurotypical people often struggle to understand neurodivergent communication styles just as much as neurodivergent people struggle to understand neurotypical ones. It's a two-way street.

Imagine two people trying to shake hands, but one expects a firm grip and the other expects a gentle touch. Neither is wrong, but their differing expectations create an awkward interaction. The Double Empathy Problem encourages us to see these differences as distinct communication styles, each valid, rather than one being "correct" and the other "incorrect." This shift promotes **mutual understanding** over "fixing" anyone. It opens the door to creating shared communication spaces where both neurotypes can feel heard and understood.

This means that instead of thinking, "How can I help my AuDHD child understand me better?" you might also ask, "How can I adjust my communication so my AuDHD child understands *me* better?" It's about shared responsibility and a willingness to meet in the middle.

Speaking Your Truth: Communicating Needs and Boundaries

Learning to articulate your needs and boundaries as an AuDHD individual is a powerful step toward healthier relationships. This can be challenging, especially if you're used to masking or suppressing your natural ways of being. But remember, your needs are valid, and communicating them clearly is a form of self-respect.

Here are some practical scripts and frameworks for communicating needs and boundaries to neurotypical loved ones:

1. **Be Direct and Specific:** Don't hint. Say exactly what you need.

    - *Instead of:* "I'm feeling overwhelmed by all the noise."

    - *Try:* "**I need to go to a quiet room for 15 minutes to reset.** My senses are overloaded."

    - *Instead of:* "I'm not sure I can handle that right now."

    - *Try:* "**I can do X, but Y is too much for me today.** Can we split it up?"

2. **Use "I" Statements:** Focus on your experience without blaming the other person.

   - *Instead of:* "You always talk too fast."

   - *Try:* "**I find it hard to process information when it comes quickly.** Could you please slow down a little?"

   - *Instead of:* "You never understand what I mean."

   - *Try:* "**I feel misunderstood when I try to explain things, and I think it's because our communication styles are different.** How can we make sure we're on the same page?"

3. **Explain the "Why" (Briefly):** Providing context can help others understand, but don't feel you need to over-explain or justify yourself.

   - *Scenario:* You need a predictable schedule.

   - *Script:* "**I thrive on routine, so knowing the plan helps me manage my energy and anxiety.** Could we try to set a consistent time for X each week?"

   - *Scenario:* You struggle with unexpected social visits.

   - *Script:* "**My brain needs time to prepare for social interactions.** Please text me an hour before you plan to drop by so I can get ready."

4. **Offer Solutions or Alternatives:** This shows you're willing to work together.

- o *Scenario:* You find large social gatherings overwhelming.

- o *Script:* "**Big parties are really draining for me, but I'd love to see you.** How about we meet for coffee next week, just the two of us?"

- o *Scenario:* You prefer written instructions.

- o *Script:* "**I process written information best.** Could you send me the details for that task in an email after we talk?"

5. **Set Clear Boundaries with Kindness but Firmness:**

- o *Script:* "**I need to stop this conversation now because I'm getting overwhelmed.** We can pick it up later when I've had a chance to calm down."

- o *Script:* "**I love you, and I want to spend time together, but I need some quiet alone time every day to recharge.** This helps me be my best self with you."

Remember, communicating your needs and boundaries isn't about being difficult; it's about creating an environment where you can both flourish. It takes practice and patience, but the payoff—more authentic connections and less misunderstanding—is well worth the effort. By speaking your truth, you invite others to meet you where you are, fostering truly empathetic and practical communication.

Key Takeaways

- Communication differences in AuDHD individuals are about distinct styles, not deficits. Challenges can include conversational flow, interpreting social cues, and understanding tone.

- Strategies for clearer communication include **avoiding subtext**, offering **explicit explanations**, and **using written communication** for important details.

- The **Double Empathy Problem** highlights mutual misunderstanding between neurotypes, shifting focus from "fixing" to fostering mutual understanding.

- Communicating needs and boundaries effectively means being **direct and specific**, using **"I" statements**, briefly explaining the **"why"**, offering **solutions**, and setting **clear boundaries** with kindness.

Chapter 6: Building Your Support System

Friends, Family & Community

Feeling alone can be a heavy burden, especially when you navigate the world with a unique brain setup like AuDHD. It's like trying to find your way through a maze without a map, and sometimes, it seems no one else understands the twists and turns you're experiencing. But here's the hopeful truth: you don't have to go it alone. Building a strong support system—whether it's with friends, family, or a wider community—is not just helpful; it's truly essential. It gives you a place to land, a space to be truly yourself, and people who can genuinely see and appreciate your strengths while understanding your challenges. This section will guide you on how to create those vital connections, turning potential isolation into a powerful network of understanding and shared experience.

Educating Your Loved Ones About AuDHD

One of the most impactful things you can do for your relationships is to help your loved ones understand what AuDHD actually is. It's not always easy, as there's a lot of misinformation out there. But remember, most people want to support you; they just might not know how. Providing them with accurate, easy-to-digest information can bridge a great divide.

Start by explaining that AuDHD isn't just "a bit of this" and "a bit of that." It's a **neurotype**, meaning your brain is wired differently from a neurotypical brain. This wiring influences everything from how you process sensory input (loud noises, bright lights) to how you think, feel, and communicate.

When talking to family and friends, focus on how AuDHD shows up *for you*. Give them concrete examples. For instance, you might say:

- "When I get overwhelmed by too much conversation or noise, it's not because I don't want to be with you. It's like my brain's processing system gets flooded, and I need quiet to reset. It's not a choice; it's a sensory response."

- "My difficulty with eye contact isn't a sign of disrespect or disinterest. For me, looking into someone's eyes while trying to listen to their words is like trying to read two books at once. It makes it harder to focus on what you're saying."

- "Sometimes I might miss social cues, like if you're upset or hinting at something. My brain tends to take things very literally. So, it really helps me if you can be direct and say exactly what you mean."

- "My 'hyperfocus' on certain interests isn't just a hobby; it's how my brain engages deeply. It's a source of joy and energy for me. And the ADHD part means I might jump between interests, which can look scattered, but it's part of my creative process."

You could also share reliable resources with them. This might include articles, books, or reputable online communities. Suggest they watch documentaries or listen to podcasts by AuDHD individuals who share their experiences. Make it clear that this isn't about them "fixing" you, but about them gaining a better grasp of your internal world.

Consider an example: David, an AuDHD man, found his sister, Sarah, often got frustrated when he'd interrupt her stories or jump between topics. David explained to her, "My brain sometimes moves really fast, and when an idea pops up, I blurt it out before I lose it. It's part of my ADHD, and it's not meant to be rude. I'm actually trying to stay engaged. Could you gently remind me to let you finish, and I'll work on it?" Sarah appreciated the explanation and felt less personally attacked. She started using a gentle hand signal to indicate when she wanted to finish her thought, and their communication improved immensely.

Finding Your Neurokin: Connecting with Others Like You

One of the most validating experiences you can have is connecting with other AuDHD individuals, or your **"neurokin."** These are people who just *get it* without you having to explain yourself constantly. This shared understanding can be a huge source of relief and strength.

There are many ways to find your neurokin:

1. **Online Support Groups:** The internet offers a wealth of communities. Look for Facebook groups, Reddit forums, or Discord servers specifically for AuDHD individuals. These spaces allow you to connect with people globally, share experiences, ask questions, and offer support. Just remember to find groups that are well-moderated and focus on positive, validating interactions.

2. **In-Person Support Groups:** While less common than online groups, some areas have local meet-ups for

neurodivergent individuals. Check with local autism or ADHD associations, community centers, or mental health organizations. These can provide a wonderful opportunity for face-to-face connection, which some people prefer.

3. **Social Media Hashtags:** Explore platforms like Instagram, TikTok, and Twitter using hashtags like #AuDHD, #neurodivergent, #autisticADHD, and #ADHDautism. Many AuDHD creators share their experiences, and you can connect with others in their comments sections or through direct messages.

4. **Neurodivergent-Affirming Therapists or Coaches:** If you're working with a therapist or coach who specializes in neurodiversity, they might be able to connect you with local resources or groups.

5. **Special Interest Groups:** Sometimes, you'll find your neurokin in groups dedicated to your specific interests, regardless of whether they're explicitly AuDHD. The shared passion often creates a welcoming environment where neurodivergent traits are accepted or even celebrated.

When you find these connections, you'll discover a common language, shared humor, and a sense that you're not an anomaly, but rather part of a unique and wonderful community. It's like finding missing pieces of your personal puzzle.

Blending Comfort and Closeness: Intimate Relationships

Intimate relationships, whether romantic or deep friendships, bring their own set of joys and challenges for AuDHD individuals. The desire for closeness often coexists with a profound need for comfort, predictability, and sometimes, a lot of alone time. This can feel like a contradiction to partners who expect constant togetherness or spontaneous adventures.

The key here is **open and honest communication about needs.** Your partner needs to understand that your need for solitude isn't a rejection of them. It's a way you regulate your nervous system and recharge your social batteries. Similarly, your desire for routine or specific sensory environments isn't about being rigid; it's about creating a safe and predictable foundation that allows you to thrive.

Transforming misunderstandings into opportunities for teamwork is a truly powerful approach. Instead of letting a miscommunication fester, view it as a chance for both of you to learn more about each other's operating systems.

Consider Emma and Liam. Emma (AuDHD) loves spending evenings at home, reading, and engaging in her special interests. Liam, her neurotypical partner, initially felt neglected when Emma often declined going out. They sat down and talked. Emma explained that her evenings at home were crucial for her energy regulation and sensory comfort. Liam, in turn, expressed his need for shared experiences outside the home. They came up with a plan: two nights a week, they would do an activity Liam enjoyed, like going to a quiet restaurant or a movie, and the other nights, Emma would have her quiet time. On those quiet nights, they might still cuddle on the couch or briefly connect, respecting Emma's need for calm. This wasn't about compromise as much as it was about creating a system that worked for both their needs.

Here's how to foster this teamwork:

- **Schedule "Together Alone" Time:** This is time spent in the same space but doing separate, calming activities. For example, you might be reading while your partner watches TV in the same room. It fulfills the need for proximity without the pressure of active social engagement.

- **Create Shared Routines:** Establish predictable routines for daily life, chores, and even leisure activities. Predictability can greatly reduce anxiety and free up mental energy.

- **Discuss Sensory Needs Explicitly:** Talk about what sensory input is comforting or overwhelming. This might involve dimming lights, using headphones, or choosing quiet environments for dates.

- **Practice "Check-Ins":** Regularly check in with each other about how you're both feeling and what you need. This could be a quick text during the day or a brief conversation in the evening.

- **Remember the 80/20 Rule (or something similar):** Not every interaction will be perfectly smooth, and that's fine. If 80% of your communication and interactions are positive and understood, that's a huge success. Focus on the overall pattern of support and effort.

Community and Validation: Overcoming Isolation

Isolation is a common struggle for many AuDHD individuals. The energy required to mask, the frequent misunderstandings, and the feeling of being "different" can lead to withdrawing from social situations. But validation— the feeling of being seen, heard, and accepted for who you are—is a fundamental human need. Finding a community that offers this can truly change your life.

Being part of a community of neurokin provides:

- **Affirmation:** When you share an experience and someone says, "Me too! I thought I was the only one," it's incredibly powerful. It confirms that your experiences are valid and shared.

- **Shared Strategies:** You can learn practical tips and coping mechanisms from others who face similar challenges.

- **Reduced Masking:** In these spaces, you often feel safe enough to unmask, to be your authentic self without fear of judgment. This reduces mental fatigue and allows for genuine connection.

- **Advocacy and Support:** Communities can band together to advocate for better understanding, accommodations, and support in wider society.

Building robust and supportive networks takes effort, but it's a journey worth taking.

Actionable Steps for Building Your Network

1. **Identify Your Needs:** What kind of support are you looking for? Do you need practical advice, emotional validation, or simply a place to vent? Knowing your needs will help you find the right groups.

2. **Start Small:** You don't have to join every group or attend every event. Begin with one online forum or one local meet-up. See how it feels.

3. **Be Patient:** Finding your people takes time. Don't get discouraged if the first group isn't the perfect fit. Keep exploring.

4. **Engage Authentically:** Once you find a space you like, participate! Share your experiences, ask questions, and offer support to others. The more you put in, the more you'll get out.

5. **Set Boundaries:** Even in supportive communities, it's important to protect your energy. Don't feel obligated to respond to every message or attend every gathering if you're feeling overwhelmed.

6. **Educate Your Allies:** For your neurotypical friends and family who are genuinely trying to understand, educate them. Share articles, explain your experiences, and guide them on how they can best support you. They can be invaluable allies in your network.

Building a strong network of friends, family, and neurokin provides a safety net and a springboard. It's a place where you can celebrate your uniqueness, learn from others, and feel truly at home in your own skin. This connection counters the isolating nature that AuDHD can sometimes present, leading to a life rich with understanding and acceptance.

Key Takeaways

- Educating loved ones about AuDHD through **specific examples** and reliable resources can greatly improve understanding in relationships.

- Connecting with **"neurokin"** through online and in-person groups provides vital validation, shared strategies, and a space to unmask.

- In intimate relationships, **open communication about needs** (like for solitude or routine) and turning misunderstandings into **opportunities for teamwork** helps blend comfort with closeness.

- Building a strong community is essential to counter isolation, offering **affirmation, shared strategies, reduced masking**, and overall **validation**.

A Thought on Moving Forward

Life has its own unique rhythm for each of us, and for those with AuDHD, that rhythm might feel a little different from the mainstream. But different doesn't mean less. It simply means a unique way of experiencing, interacting, and contributing to the world. By embracing clarity in communication, seeking out your true community, and building bridges of understanding with those you hold dear, you're not just navigating challenges; you're creating a life that is authentic, fulfilling, and truly your own. The journey may have its unexpected detours, but with the right tools and the right company, every step can be a step toward a deeper, more genuine connection.

Chapter 7: AuDHD in the Workplace

Accommodations & Career Paths

Working can be a big part of life, taking up a lot of our time and energy. For someone with AuDHD, traditional workplaces can feel like trying to fit a square peg into a round hole. The usual office hum, the constant interruptions, or the unspoken rules can be more than just annoying; they can be truly draining, sometimes leading to burnout. But here's the good news: with some practical approaches, you can make work work *for you*. This part of our discussion will show you how to find your place in the working world, making it a space where your unique abilities can shine, not dim.

Imagine trying to do your best work while a jackhammer is going off outside your window, and someone keeps tapping you on the shoulder every five minutes to ask a quick question. That's a bit like what a typical workday can feel like for many AuDHD individuals. The sensory input, the constant shifting of attention, and the unwritten social rules of the office can stack up, making it hard to focus, be productive, and simply feel comfortable. The challenges are real, but so are the ways to make things better. This chapter aims to give you the practical steps to advocate for yourself and craft a career that brings out your best.

Challenges in Traditional Work Environments

Traditional workplaces often operate on assumptions that don't always align with the needs of an AuDHD brain. These can be the source of significant friction and stress.

First, think about **sensory overload**. Open-plan offices, a common setup these days, can be a nightmare. The constant chatter, the ringing phones, the clacking keyboards, the flickering fluorescent lights—it all combines into a cacophony that can make concentrating nearly impossible. For someone with heightened sensory sensitivities, this isn't just distracting; it's physically uncomfortable and exhausting. This constant bombardment leads to sensory overwhelm, making it hard to think clearly or regulate emotions.

Next, consider the demands on **attention and focus**. ADHD often means a struggle with sustained attention on tasks that aren't inherently interesting, alongside a tendency to be easily distracted. Autism often brings a preference for routine and focused work without interruption. Put them together, and you might find it hard to start a task, get pulled off track by minor stimuli, and then struggle to switch back to the original task. This can make meeting deadlines or managing multiple projects a constant uphill battle.

Then there are **social dynamics**. Workplace culture often relies on unspoken expectations, subtle cues, and a lot of informal communication. Water cooler chats, office politics, and interpreting sarcasm or indirect feedback can be confusing and draining for AuDHD individuals. You might miss a social cue that's obvious to everyone else, or you might unintentionally say something that's taken the wrong way, not because you meant to, but because your communication style is direct. This can lead to feeling isolated or misunderstood by colleagues and managers.

For instance, consider Alex, an AuDHD software developer. He worked in a busy, open-plan office. The constant noise and interruptions made it almost impossible for him to get into a state of **hyperfocus**, which is where he did his best

51

coding. He would often put on headphones, but colleagues would still tap his shoulder for "quick questions." Alex also found the informal team lunches overwhelming, preferring to eat alone, which led some colleagues to label him as "antisocial." He was brilliant at his job when he could focus, but the environment was chipping away at his well-being and productivity.

Disclosing Your Diagnosis and Requesting Accommodations

Deciding to disclose your AuDHD diagnosis at work is a personal choice. There's no single "right" way to do it, and it depends on your workplace culture, your relationship with your manager, and your own comfort level. However, understanding your rights and how to ask for **accommodations** can make a huge difference in your success and comfort.

If you choose to disclose, it's often best to do so with your direct manager or someone in Human Resources (HR). Focus on what you need to do your job well, rather than just stating your diagnosis. Frame your requests around how they will help you be a more effective employee.

Here's a general framework for requesting accommodations:

1. **Educate Yourself:** Know your rights under disability laws in your region (e.g., the Americans with Disabilities Act in the U.S.). This helps you understand what constitutes a "reasonable accommodation."

2. **Identify Your Specific Needs:** Before you talk to anyone, make a list of the challenges you face at work due to your AuDHD. Then, think about concrete solutions or changes that would help.

52

- Do you need a quiet space?

- Do you need instructions in writing?

- Do you need flexible hours to manage energy levels or appointments?

- Do you need to use noise-canceling headphones?

3. **Prepare Your Request:** Write down what you plan to say. It helps to keep it clear and to the point. You might say something like, "I'm sharing with you that I have AuDHD, and this impacts me in X, Y, and Z ways at work. To do my best work, I would benefit from the following accommodations."

4. **Propose Solutions:** Instead of just listing problems, offer solutions. For example:

   - **Flexible hours:** "I find that my most productive hours are early mornings or late afternoons. Could I adjust my schedule to start at 7 AM and leave at 3 PM, as long as I complete my required hours?"

   - **Quiet workspace:** "The noise in the open office makes it difficult for me to concentrate. Could I work from home X days a week, or could I have a desk in a quieter area or a small office?"

   - **Clear instructions:** "I process information best when it's given to me in writing, with clear steps. Could you please send me follow-up emails after meetings with action items, or provide project briefs in a written format?"

- **Use of noise-canceling headphones:** "To help me focus in the open office, I find that using noise-canceling headphones is very effective. Would it be okay for me to use these throughout the day?"

- **Scheduled breaks:** "I need regular short breaks to prevent sensory overload and maintain focus. Could I take a 10-minute break every hour?"

5. **Be Ready for Discussion:** Your employer might have questions or suggest alternative solutions. Be open to discussing options that meet both your needs and the business's requirements.

6. **Document Everything:** Keep a record of your discussions, requests, and any agreements made. This protects both you and your employer.

For example, Sarah, a graphic designer with AuDHD, found the constant "pop-in" interruptions from colleagues at her cubicle disruptive. She approached her manager, explaining, "I really enjoy my work here, and I want to be as productive as possible. I find that when I'm in the middle of a design, unexpected interruptions make it very hard to get back into my flow. To help me maintain my focus, would it be possible for colleagues to message me on our internal chat system before coming over, or for me to put up a 'do not disturb' sign when I'm working on something that needs deep concentration?" Her manager, seeing Sarah's commitment to her work, agreed to the suggestions, and Sarah's productivity—and stress levels—improved significantly.

Leveraging AuDHD Strengths in Professional Settings

While there are challenges, AuDHD also brings a suite of powerful strengths that can make you an exceptional employee. Recognizing and leaning into these can open doors to incredibly fulfilling career paths.

1. **Creative Problem-Solving:** The autistic mind often sees patterns and connections that others miss, while ADHD thinking can lead to brainstorming many diverse solutions quickly. This combination can lead to highly original and effective ways to solve problems. You might approach a challenge from an unexpected angle, finding a simpler or more innovative answer.

2. **Attention to Detail:** Many AuDHD individuals possess a remarkable ability to notice fine details that others overlook. This can be invaluable in roles requiring precision, quality control, or meticulous analysis. It's like having a built-in magnifying glass for specifics.

3. **Hyperfocus:** When an AuDHD individual is truly interested in a task, they can enter a state of **hyperfocus**, where they become completely absorbed, ignoring distractions and working for extended periods with intense concentration. This allows for deep, high-quality work to be done efficiently.

4. **Unique Perspectives:** Because your brain processes information differently, you often bring fresh, unconventional viewpoints to discussions. This can lead to innovative ideas, spotting potential issues, or simplifying complex systems in ways neurotypical individuals might not consider.

5. **Strong Sense of Justice and Integrity:** Many AuDHD individuals have a deep commitment to fairness and honesty. This can make them highly trustworthy and ethical employees who stand up for what's right.

6. **Persistence (in areas of interest):** When engaged in a special interest or a task that aligns with their passion, AuDHD individuals can exhibit incredible persistence, working tirelessly to achieve mastery or complete a project.

Consider Maria, an AuDHD woman working as a data analyst. Her colleagues marveled at her ability to spot tiny discrepancies in vast datasets that everyone else missed. This was her **attention to detail** and pattern recognition at play. When a new, complex database needed organizing, Maria entered a state of **hyperfocus**, working for hours on end, meticulously structuring the data. She also suggested a new, more logical way to categorize certain information, something no one else had thought of, demonstrating her **unique perspective** and creative problem-solving. Maria's manager quickly learned to give her tasks that aligned with her strengths, making her an indispensable part of the team.

Finding Work That Aligns with Special Interests

One of the most effective ways to prevent burnout and maximize your strengths as an AuDHD individual is to find work that genuinely aligns with your **special interests**. When your job involves something you're naturally passionate about, it taps into your intrinsic motivation, makes **hyperfocus** more accessible, and reduces the mental load of forcing yourself to care about something uninteresting.

Think about careers that allow for:

- **Deep Specialization:** Roles where you can become an expert in a specific niche. This could be in research, highly technical fields (like software engineering, data science, specific types of engineering), archiving, or curatorial work.

- **Structured and Predictable Environments:** Some AuDHD individuals thrive in environments with clear rules, predictable tasks, and minimal unexpected changes. Consider roles in quality assurance, library science, certain types of accounting, or laboratory work.

- **Problem-Solving Focus:** Careers that allow you to constantly tackle new and interesting problems, such as certain areas of IT, scientific research, or forensic analysis.

- **Creative Expression:** If your special interests lean artistic, look for roles in design, writing, music, or crafting that allow for focused, detailed work.

- **Independent Work:** Many AuDHD individuals prefer working alone or with minimal social interaction. Freelancing, remote work, or roles that involve independent project completion can be a good fit.

For example, Mark, who has AuDHD, found traditional office jobs stifling. He had a lifelong special interest in vintage electronics and spent his free time repairing old radios and record players. He decided to turn this passion into a career. He started a small business repairing and restoring antique electronics from his home workshop. The work allowed him to **hyperfocus** on intricate details, learn continuously about his passion, and control his work environment to minimize sensory input. He was able to set his own hours, manage client interactions on his terms, and genuinely enjoy his work, avoiding the burnout he experienced in previous jobs.

The path to a fulfilling career as an AuDHD individual might look different from the traditional route, and that's perfectly fine. It's about empowering yourself to advocate for what you need and strategically finding or creating environments where your unique talents can truly flourish. Your AuDHD isn't a barrier to a great career; it's a map to one that suits you perfectly.

Key Takeaways

- Traditional workplaces pose challenges for AuDHD individuals due to **sensory overload**, difficulties with **attention and focus**, and complex **social dynamics**.

- When disclosing a diagnosis, **focus on specific needs** and propose **concrete solutions** for accommodations like flexible hours, quiet spaces, clear instructions, and using noise-canceling headphones.

- AuDHD strengths, such as **creative problem-solving, attention to detail, hyperfocus**, and **unique perspectives**, can be leveraged to excel professionally.

- Seeking careers that **align with special interests** helps prevent burnout and maximizes natural talents, leading to more fulfilling work experiences.

Chapter 8:Education Strategies for AuDHD Adults

Learning doesn't stop after school ends; it's a lifelong process, especially for adults with AuDHD. Whether you're considering going back to college, starting a vocational training program, or simply learning a new skill for personal enjoyment or career growth, the way you approach learning matters a great deal. The traditional classroom or study methods might not always fit how your brain works, and that's okay. This chapter will give you practical guidance on how to make learning an effective and enjoyable experience, tailored to your specific needs as an AuDHD adult. It's about adapting the learning environment to you, not the other way around.

Effective Learning Strategies for AuDHD Adults

Navigating higher education or vocational training with AuDHD can bring its own set of hurdles, but with the right strategies, you can truly shine. The key is to recognize how your brain learns best and then to actively create those conditions for yourself.

One highly effective strategy is **multimodal instruction**. This means learning through various senses and methods. If you're in a class, don't just listen to the lecture. Also, take notes (typing or writing), draw diagrams, or use flashcards. If a topic is discussed verbally, try to find a video about it, read an article, or even explain it out loud to yourself. Different pathways to the same information can help it stick better and address the varying ways your AuDHD brain processes data. For example, if you are learning about history, watching a documentary, reading a historical fiction book, and visiting a museum exhibit can all combine to create a richer learning experience than just reading a textbook.

Another crucial technique is **breaking down large assignments**. The thought of a huge research paper or a multi-part project can feel overwhelming, triggering procrastination or paralysis. Instead, divide these big tasks into smaller, manageable chunks. Think of each chunk as a mini-assignment with its own small deadline. For instance, a research paper could be broken down into:

1. Choose topic and preliminary research (Day 1-2).

2. Create an outline (Day 3).

3. Write introduction (Day 4).

4. Write body paragraph 1 (Day 5).

5. And so on. This approach makes the task seem less daunting and gives you a sense of accomplishment with each completed step, helping to maintain motivation.

Requesting extra time for tasks is not a sign of weakness; it's a legitimate accommodation that can dramatically reduce stress and improve your performance. If you're in a formal educational setting, most institutions have disability services offices that can grant this. Explain that due to your AuDHD, you sometimes need more time to process information, organize thoughts, or manage sensory overwhelm that might interfere with concentration. Don't wait until the last minute to ask; make this request early in your course or program.

Utilizing quiet study spaces is also incredibly important. Just like in the workplace, sensory distractions can derail your focus. Seek out libraries, quiet corners of a coffee shop (with headphones!), or a dedicated space at home where you can minimize noise and visual clutter. For some, a perfectly silent room might be too much, and a gentle white noise machine or instrumental music could be helpful. Experiment to find what works best for you.

Think about a student, Leo, who decided to go back to college for a new career path. He found it hard to sit through long lectures and felt anxious about upcoming exams. He spoke to the disability services office and arranged for accommodations: he was allowed to record lectures (so he could listen back at his own pace), he received extended time on tests, and he was given access to a quiet room for exams. In his personal study, he used noise-canceling headphones and broke his reading assignments into 30-minute chunks with 5-minute movement breaks. These adjustments helped him go from struggling to excelling.

Continuous Learning for Neurodivergent Brains

The idea that learning stops after you get a degree or a certificate is outdated. For AuDHD adults, **continuous learning and skill development** are not just career boosters; they can be sources of deep satisfaction and engagement. Your brain thrives on novelty and deep interest.

Here's why ongoing learning is so powerful for AuDHD individuals:

- **Taps into Special Interests:** This is where you truly shine. Learning about a topic you're passionate about doesn't feel like work. It feels like exploration. If you can align your learning with your special interests, you'll find it energizing rather than draining.

- **Provides Structure and Routine:** Structured learning can provide a sense of purpose and routine, which many AuDHD individuals benefit from. This could be signing up for an online course, joining a workshop series, or committing to a regular study schedule.

- **Keeps the Brain Engaged:** The ADHD side of AuDHD often craves new stimulation. Continuous learning provides this in a constructive way, helping to avoid boredom and restlessness.

- **Builds Mastery:** The autistic aspect often drives a desire for deep knowledge and mastery. Learning new skills allows you to pursue this drive, gaining expertise that can be personally rewarding and professionally valuable.

Consider Sarah, an AuDHD accountant who felt her job was becoming monotonous. She had a special interest in coding and data visualization. Even though it wasn't directly related to her day job, she enrolled in an online course for Python programming, dedicating an hour each evening to it. This allowed her to **hyperfocus** on something she found deeply engaging, reducing her workday stress and providing a creative outlet. Eventually, she was able to apply her new coding skills to automate some of her accounting tasks, making her more efficient at work and opening new career opportunities.

Actionable Advice for Adult Learners

1. **Know Your Learning Style:** Are you visual, auditory, kinesthetic? Many AuDHD individuals are highly visual or kinesthetic. Experiment with different methods:

- Visual: Use diagrams, mind maps, color-coding, flashcards with images.

- Auditory: Listen to lectures, podcasts, or record yourself explaining concepts.

- Kinesthetic: Pace while you study, use fidget toys, write notes by hand, or act out concepts.

2. **Use Technology Wisely:**

   - **Task Management Apps:** Use apps like Todoist or Trello to break down tasks and track progress.

   - **Reminders/Alarms:** Set alarms for study breaks, deadlines, or to switch tasks.

   - **Text-to-Speech/Speech-to-Text:** If reading or typing is difficult, use these tools to process information differently or to get your thoughts down.

   - **Noise-Canceling Apps/Headphones:** Block out distractions.

3. **Create a Dedicated Study Environment:** This doesn't have to be a whole room, just a specific, consistent spot where you do your learning. Keep it organized and free of unnecessary clutter.

4. **Incorporate Movement:** Don't sit still for too long. Take short walks, stretch, or do some light exercise during breaks to help your brain reset and absorb information.

5. **Be Your Own Advocate:** Don't hesitate to ask instructors, tutors, or support staff for

accommodations or clarification. They are there to help.

6. **Find a Study Buddy (or a Body Doubling Partner):** Sometimes, just having another person present (even if you're working on separate things) can help with focus and motivation, a concept known as "body doubling."

7. **Prioritize Self-Care:** Learning can be mentally demanding. Make sure you're getting enough sleep, eating nourishing foods, and taking genuine breaks to prevent burnout. Your brain works best when it's well-rested and cared for.

8. **Embrace Your Interests:** If you find a topic that sparks your **hyperfocus**, lean into it! This is where your most intense and satisfying learning will happen. Don't force yourself to learn things that utterly bore you if you have a choice.

The journey of learning for an AuDHD adult is a continuous one, full of potential for deep connection with subjects you love and growth in areas you want to master. By recognizing your unique learning style and applying practical strategies, you can turn any learning challenge into an exciting opportunity. This approach helps you not only acquire knowledge but also to genuinely thrive in your intellectual pursuits.

Key Takeaways

- AuDHD adults benefit from **multimodal instruction, breaking down large assignments**, requesting **extra**

time, and utilizing **quiet study spaces** in educational settings.

- **Continuous learning** is important for neurodivergent brains, tapping into special interests and providing structure and mental engagement.

- Actionable advice includes **knowing your learning style, using technology wisely** for organization and focus, creating a **dedicated study environment**, incorporating **movement, advocating for yourself**, considering a **study buddy**, and prioritizing **self-care**.

A Concluding Reflection

It's clear that living with AuDHD means experiencing the world with a unique lens—one that brings both distinct challenges and truly remarkable strengths. Whether it's finding your footing in the workplace or continuing to learn and grow, the aim is not to change who you are, but to create environments and strategies that allow your authentic self to flourish. By understanding your own operating system, advocating for your needs, and leaning into your natural abilities, you can build a life that feels not just manageable, but genuinely rich and rewarding. The journey is yours, and with these practical steps, you're well-equipped to navigate it with confidence and hope.

Chapter 9: Emotional Regulation

Navigating Intense Feelings

Feelings—we all have them, sometimes a whole rollercoaster of them. For someone with AuDHD, these feelings can feel extra intense, extra loud, or extra confusing. It's like having the volume turned up on your emotions, and sometimes, the dial seems stuck. This can lead to moments where things feel truly overwhelming, where a small trigger can set off a big reaction. But here's the hopeful part: you are not at the mercy of these intense feelings. Just like you can learn to play an instrument or ride a bike, you can learn ways to navigate your emotional world with more calm and control. This section offers practical approaches to help you understand and manage your feelings, turning that emotional rollercoaster into a much smoother ride.

Emotional dysregulation—it's a mouthful, isn't it? But for many AuDHD individuals, it's a very real experience. This means that your feelings can come on strong, shift quickly, and sometimes feel impossible to manage. Small frustrations can become huge waves of anger, mild discomfort can turn into deep distress, or sensory input can trigger an overwhelming emotional response. This isn't a flaw in your character; it's a difference in how your brain processes emotions and external stimuli. Understanding this is the first step toward gaining more control and peace.

Think of your emotional system like a finely tuned instrument. For someone AuDHD, that instrument might be more sensitive to vibrations, leading to bigger, louder notes when a neurotypical person's instrument might just hum gently. The goal isn't to get rid of the instrument, but to learn how to play it with more skill and harmony.

Understanding Emotional Dysregulation in AuDHD

So, what exactly makes emotions feel so intense for AuDHD individuals? It's often a combination of factors related to both autism and ADHD characteristics.

One aspect is **sensory overload**. If your system is constantly bombarded by too much noise, light, touch, or even too many conversations, your overall stress level stays high. When your stress bucket is already full from sensory input, even a tiny additional stressor can make it overflow, leading to an intense emotional reaction. It's like adding a single drop of water to an already full glass—it just spills over.

Another contributing factor is **difficulty with executive functions**. ADHD often brings challenges with executive functions, which are the mental skills that help you plan, focus, remember, and manage impulses. When your executive functions are struggling, it becomes harder to:

- **Pause and think** before reacting impulsively.
- **Shift attention** away from an upsetting thought or situation.
- **Problem-solve** a way out of a frustrating situation.
- **Regulate your energy** levels, which directly impacts emotional stability.

Then there's the **alexithymia** often present in autistic individuals, which means difficulty identifying and describing emotions. You might *feel* something intensely, but not be able to name it or understand *why* you feel it. This makes it much harder to address the emotion or communicate what's happening internally, leading to frustration and a sense of being out of control.

Finally, a strong sense of **justice and fairness**, common in autism, can also contribute to intense emotional reactions. If something feels unfair or unjust, the emotional response can be powerful and overwhelming.

Consider Mark, an AuDHD man who works from home. His partner, Sarah, unexpectedly brought home a barking puppy. Mark instantly felt a surge of intense anxiety and anger. The constant, unpredictable barking was sensory torture for his autistic side, quickly overloading his system. The ADHD side made it hard for him to calm his racing thoughts or effectively plan how to address the situation. He felt overwhelmed, his chest tightened, and he yelled, "Get that dog out of here!" startling Sarah. This wasn't just about a puppy; it was about sensory overload combining with executive function challenges, leading to emotional dysregulation.

Practical Strategies for Managing Intense Emotions

The good news is that you can develop a toolkit of strategies to help you manage intense emotions. These are like tools you practice using when things are relatively calm, so they're ready when a storm hits.

1. **Mindfulness Practices:** This isn't about emptying your mind; it's about paying attention to the present moment without judgment. It helps you notice emotions as they arise, giving you a chance to respond thoughtfully rather than react impulsively.

- **Body Scan:** Lie down or sit comfortably. Gently bring your attention to different parts of your body, noticing any sensations (warmth, tension, tingling) without trying to change them. Just observe. This helps you reconnect with your physical self, which can be grounding when emotions are overwhelming.

- **Mindful Breathing:** Pay attention to your breath. Notice the feeling of air entering and leaving your body. If your mind wanders, gently bring it back to your breath. Even a few minutes can help you create space between you and your emotions.

2. **Deep Breathing Exercises:** This is a powerful, immediate tool. Slow, deep breaths activate your body's relaxation response.

- **Box Breathing (4-4-4-4):** Inhale slowly through your nose for a count of **4**. Hold your breath for a count of **4**. Exhale slowly through your mouth for a count of **4**. Hold your breath for a count of **4**. Repeat several times. This structured breathing provides a focus for your ADHD brain and calms your nervous system.

- **Diaphragmatic Breathing:** Place one hand on your chest and one on your belly. Inhale deeply, focusing on making your belly rise, not your chest. Exhale slowly, feeling your belly fall. This promotes deeper, more calming breaths.

3. **Grounding Techniques:** When you feel overwhelmed or disconnected, grounding techniques help bring your awareness back to the present moment and your physical surroundings.

   - **5-4-3-2-1 Method:**
     - Name **5** things you can see.
     - Name **4** things you can touch (and actually touch them if you can).
     - Name **3** things you can hear.
     - Name **2** things you can smell.
     - Name **1** thing you can taste.

   - **Physical Grounding:** Press your feet firmly into the floor. Feel the contact. Notice the texture of your clothes against your skin. Hold an ice cube in your hand (the intense sensation can be very redirecting). Splash cold water on your face.

4. **Emotional Labeling:** As mentioned, naming emotions can be tough. But even if you can only label it as "uncomfortable" or "tense," it's a step.

   - **Use an Emotion Wheel:** Look up an "emotion wheel" online. This chart helps you identify specific emotions by starting with broad categories and narrowing them down. This can be a useful tool when you feel a big emotion but can't quite pinpoint what it is.

   - **"I feel [emotion] because [situation]."** Practice this simple sentence. Even if the "why" isn't clear, just naming the emotion can lessen its power. For example, "I feel frustrated because this task is harder than I expected."

For instance, when Sarah (from the puppy example) felt that surge of anger and anxiety, she could have first used **box breathing** to slow her racing heart. Then, she might have used the **5-4-3-2-1 grounding technique** to bring herself back to the room. After a few minutes, when she felt a tiny bit calmer, she could try **emotional labeling**: "I feel overwhelmed and angry because the barking is hurting my ears and it was unexpected." This wouldn't solve the puppy situation, but it would prevent the immediate explosion and allow her to approach the problem more calmly.

Preventing and Recovering from Meltdowns and Shutdowns

Meltdowns and shutdowns are intense reactions to overwhelm, often specific to autistic individuals (and by extension, AuDHD individuals). They are not temper tantrums. A **meltdown** is an externalized, explosive response to overload, while a **shutdown** is an internalized, withdrawal response. Both are signs that your system has reached its limit.

Preventing Meltdowns and Shutdowns:

1. **Identify Your Triggers:** What consistently leads to overwhelm for you? Is it loud noises, unexpected changes, too much social interaction, bright lights, specific foods, or certain smells? Keep a **"trigger log"** for a week or two.

2. **Monitor Your "Stress Bucket":** Imagine you have a bucket that fills up with all the stressors of the day—

sensory input, social demands, executive function challenges, unexpected changes. When it gets too full, a meltdown or shutdown is likely. Learn to recognize the early warning signs that your bucket is filling: irritability, increased stimming (repetitive movements or sounds), feeling fidgety, headaches, or a general sense of unease.

3. **Build in Sensory Breaks:** Proactively schedule time away from sensory input. This might mean:

   o Stepping into a quiet room for 5-10 minutes every hour.

   o Wearing noise-canceling headphones even when it's not loud.

   o Taking a walk in nature.

   o Engaging in a calming special interest.

4. **Prioritize Predictability:** Where possible, stick to routines. Knowing what to expect reduces anxiety. If a change is coming, prepare for it in advance.

5. **Communicate Your Needs Early:** If you're starting to feel overwhelmed, let loved ones or colleagues know. "I'm starting to feel a bit overwhelmed right now, I need some quiet time."

Recovering from Meltdowns and Shutdowns:

1. **Seek a Safe Space:** The most important thing is to remove yourself from the overstimulating environment if possible. Find a quiet, low-sensory space where you feel safe.

2. **Reduce Sensory Input:** Dim the lights, turn off sounds, remove uncomfortable clothing.

3. **Use Calming Sensory Input:** This might be a weighted blanket, soft music (if sensory-seeking), a warm bath, or engaging in gentle stimming.

4. **Allow Time and Space:** Do not try to rationalize, problem-solve, or push through the feelings. Your system needs to reset. This could take minutes, hours, or even a full day.

5. **Hydrate and Nourish:** Once able, drink water and have a gentle snack. Your body has used a lot of energy.

6. **Self-Compassion:** Do not blame yourself. Meltdowns and shutdowns are not failures; they are physiological responses to overwhelm. Treat yourself with the same kindness you would offer a friend.

7. **Reflect (Later):** Once you are fully recovered, gently reflect on what happened. What were the triggers? What were the warning signs? What could you do differently next time? This is for learning, not for self-criticism.

For example, Emily, an AuDHD teenager, usually loved going to her friend's house. But one day, her friend decided to have a spontaneous party with loud music, flashing lights, and many unfamiliar people. Emily felt her "stress bucket" filling rapidly. Her early warning signs were fidgeting more and feeling irritable. Instead of pushing through, which usually led to a meltdown, she remembered her strategies. She went to her friend and quietly said, "I'm getting really overwhelmed by the noise and crowds. I need to go home now." She then went to a quiet bedroom, put on her noise-canceling headphones, and pulled her weighted blanket over herself. This allowed her to enter a shutdown state where she could slowly recover, rather than erupting into an uncontrollable meltdown. This self-awareness and proactive approach made a huge difference.

Managing intense emotions is a daily practice, not a one-time fix. But with these tangible tools and a growing understanding of your own emotional landscape, you can stabilize your emotional experiences, cultivate greater inner peace, and navigate life's ups and downs with more grace.

Key Takeaways

- **Emotional dysregulation** in AuDHD stems from sensory overload, executive function challenges, alexithymia, and a strong sense of justice.

- Practice **mindfulness** (body scans, mindful breathing), **deep breathing** (box breathing, diaphragmatic breathing), and **grounding techniques** (5-4-3-2-1, physical contact) to manage intense emotions.

- **Emotional labeling** using tools like an emotion wheel helps identify and reduce the power of feelings.

- To **prevent meltdowns and shutdowns**, identify triggers, monitor your "stress bucket," build in sensory breaks, prioritize predictability, and communicate needs early.

- To **recover from meltdowns and shutdowns**, seek a safe space, reduce sensory input, use calming input, allow time and space, hydrate, practice self-compassion, and reflect later.

Chapter 10: Holistic Self-Care

Preventing Burnout & Cultivating Joy

Taking care of yourself isn't just a nice thing to do; it's a fundamental requirement for anyone with AuDHD. Often, the world pushes us to keep going, to "power through," but for a neurodivergent brain, this can lead straight to burnout. Burnout isn't just feeling tired; it's a state of emotional, physical, and mental exhaustion caused by prolonged or excessive stress. For AuDHD individuals, it's a particularly common and debilitating experience. But there's a powerful antidote: holistic self-care. This isn't a luxury; it's an indispensable strategy for managing AuDHD, protecting your well-being, and creating a life where joy isn't just a fleeting moment but a regular part of your experience.

Think of self-care as essential maintenance for your unique operating system. You wouldn't expect a high-performance car to run without the right fuel and regular servicing, would you? Your AuDHD brain is a high-performance system, and it needs consistent, tailored care to run smoothly.

Prioritizing Your Foundation: Sleep, Nutrition, and Exercise

These three pillars—sleep, nutrition, and regular exercise—are often overlooked, but they form the absolute foundation of your well-being, especially for an AuDHD brain. Neglecting any one of them can significantly impact your emotional regulation, focus, and overall energy levels.

1. **Sleep: Your Brain's Reset Button**

   o   Many AuDHD individuals struggle with sleep—either falling asleep due to a racing mind

(ADHD) or adhering to strict routines (autism). However, **consistent, quality sleep** is non-negotiable. It's when your brain cleans itself, consolidates memories, and processes emotions.

- ○ **Actionable Steps:**

    - **Establish a consistent sleep schedule:** Go to bed and wake up at roughly the same time every day, even on weekends. Your body's internal clock thrives on predictability.

    - **Create a calming bedtime routine:** This might include dimming lights, avoiding screens for an hour before bed, taking a warm bath, reading a physical book, or listening to calming music.

    - **Optimize your sleep environment:** Make sure your bedroom is dark, quiet (use earplugs or a white noise machine if needed), and cool.

    - **Consider weighted blankets:** Many AuDHD individuals find the deep pressure calming and helpful for sleep.

- ○ **Example:** Jessica, an AuDHD young adult, used to stay up late, getting caught in hyperfocus on her special interests. She always woke up exhausted and irritable. She started using a sleep tracking app and realized her sleep was inconsistent. She then implemented a strict bedtime routine: lights off at 10 PM, an hour of reading before bed, and wearing an eye mask. She also bought a weighted blanket. After a few weeks, she noticed a dramatic improvement in her daytime mood and focus.

2. **Nutrition: Fueling Your Brain**

   o What you eat directly impacts your brain function, mood, and energy. ADHD can lead to forgetfulness around meals or preference for easily accessible (often processed) foods, while autistic sensory sensitivities can make certain textures or flavors unbearable.

   o **Actionable Steps:**

      - **Focus on whole, unprocessed foods:** Lots of fruits, vegetables, lean proteins, and healthy fats.

      - **Stay hydrated:** Drink plenty of water throughout the day.

      - **Regular meal times:** Eating consistently helps regulate blood sugar, which impacts mood and concentration. Use alarms if you tend to forget meals.

      - **Prepare easy, safe foods:** Have a list of "safe" foods (foods you know you'll eat and enjoy) that are quick to prepare or grab when executive function is low.

- **Consider supplements:** After consulting with a doctor or nutritionist, some people find supplements like Omega-3s or magnesium helpful.

- **Example:** Tom, who has AuDHD, often skipped breakfast and relied on sugary snacks during the day, leading to energy crashes and irritability. He started prepping simple, high-protein breakfasts the night before (like overnight oats) and keeping a stash of healthy snacks (nuts, fruit) at his desk. This steady fuel intake significantly reduced his mood swings and helped him maintain focus throughout the workday.

3. **Regular Exercise: Moving for Mood and Focus**

   - Physical activity is a powerful tool for regulating energy, reducing anxiety, and improving mood. It helps release excess energy from ADHD and can be a predictable, repetitive activity that calms the autistic system.

   - **Actionable Steps:**

     - **Find activities you enjoy:** This is key! If it feels like a chore, you won't stick with it. This could be walking, swimming, dancing, martial arts, cycling, or even jumping on a trampoline.

     - **Incorporate movement into your day:** Take regular short breaks to stretch or walk around.

- **Aim for consistency, not intensity:** Even 15-20 minutes of moderate activity most days of the week is more beneficial than one intense workout a month.

- **Use body doubling:** Exercise with a friend or join a class for accountability if that helps.

  - **Example:** Maria, an AuDHD individual, felt constantly restless but struggled to initiate exercise. She found that long, solitary walks in a local park where she could listen to podcasts were incredibly calming and stimulating. She made it a part of her daily routine, and it became a source of both physical activity and mental quiet.

Establishing Healthy Boundaries: Preventing Overwhelm

For AuDHD individuals, the line between helpful engagement and overwhelming exhaustion can be thin. Setting **healthy boundaries** is not about being rude or selfish; it's about protecting your energy, time, and mental well-being. It's an act of self-preservation.

- **Boundary with Yourself:** This means recognizing your limits. If you're feeling overstimulated, exhausted, or emotionally drained, it's okay to say "no" to more demands, even from yourself.

  - **Example:** You have a special interest project you're hyperfocusing on, but you haven't eaten or slept properly. A boundary with yourself would be to stop for a set amount of time, eat

80

a meal, and rest, even if your brain wants to keep going.

- **Boundary with Others:** This involves communicating your needs and limits to the people around you.

  - **Time Boundaries:** "I'm available to talk until 5 PM today, then I need to focus on a project." Or, "I need to have my evenings free for quiet time."

  - **Sensory Boundaries:** "Could we meet at the quieter coffee shop?" or "I need to use my headphones during this meeting."

  - **Emotional Boundaries:** "I can't talk about that right now; I'm feeling overwhelmed." Or, "I can listen, but I can't take on your emotional problems today."

- **Actionable Steps for Setting Boundaries:**

1. **Identify your limits:** What makes you feel drained or overwhelmed?

2. **Communicate clearly and kindly:** Use "I" statements. "I need..." or "I feel overwhelmed when..."

3. **Be consistent:** The first few times you set a boundary, others might test it. Stick to your guns gently but firmly.

4. **Practice saying "no":** It's a full sentence. You don't always need a long explanation.

Finding Your Spark: Personal Interests and Creative Outlets

Engaging in your personal interests and creative outlets isn't just "fun"; it's a **powerful therapeutic tool** for emotional regulation and fostering joy. For AuDHD individuals, these activities often provide a unique blend of focused calm (autistic trait) and stimulating engagement (ADHD trait).

- **Special Interests as a Calming Anchor:** When you engage in a special interest, your brain can enter a state of **hyperfocus**, which can be incredibly regulating. It allows you to block out other stressors, feel a sense of competence, and experience deep flow. This isn't escaping reality; it's giving your brain the structured engagement it craves.

- **Creative Outlets for Expression:** Art, music, writing, crafting, coding, building—any form of creative expression—provides a way to process emotions, communicate thoughts, and find a sense of accomplishment. This can be especially important if you struggle with verbal emotional expression.

- **Actionable Steps:**
    - **Identify your passions:** What activities make you lose track of time? What topics could you talk about for hours?

    - **Schedule dedicated time:** Treat these activities like important appointments. Put them on your calendar.

    - **Protect that time:** Don't let other tasks or demands constantly encroach on your personal interest time. This is a vital part of your self-care.

- Don't worry about perfection: The goal is the process, the engagement, the joy—not necessarily a finished product. Let go of the pressure to be "good" at it.

- Example: Alex, who had difficulty with social interaction and sensory overwhelm at work, started spending his evenings building complex Lego sets. This allowed him to engage in **hyperfocus**, follow detailed instructions, and create something tangible, all in a quiet, controlled environment. This creative outlet was his go-to strategy for de-stressing and finding a sense of calm after a demanding day.

The Gentle Art of Self-Compassion and Imperfection

Perhaps the most challenging, yet most important, aspect of holistic self-care for AuDHD individuals is cultivating **self-compassion** and letting go of **perfectionistic tendencies**. Many AuDHD adults carry a lifetime of internalized criticism for not "fitting in," for making "mistakes," or for not meeting neurotypical expectations. This leads to a harsh inner critic and a drive for perfection that is both exhausting and unattainable.

- **Self-Compassion:** This means treating yourself with the same kindness, understanding, and acceptance you would offer to a dear friend who is struggling.

  - **Recognize shared humanity:** Understand that struggles are part of being human, and you're not alone in your experiences. Many AuDHD individuals feel similar things.

- **Practice mindfulness of suffering:** Acknowledge your pain or difficulty rather than ignoring or suppressing it.

- **Offer self-kindness:** Speak to yourself gently. Instead of "I'm so stupid for forgetting that," try "It's hard for my brain to remember everything, and that's okay. What can I do to help myself next time?"

- **Letting Go of Perfectionism:** The desire to do everything perfectly often leads to procrastination (fear of not being perfect) or burnout (trying too hard).

  - **"Good enough" is often enough:** Not everything needs to be perfectly polished. Sometimes, done is better than perfect.

  - **Embrace your neurodiversity:** Your brain works differently. This isn't a flaw to be perfected away; it's a unique operating system with its own strengths and challenges.

  - **Focus on progress, not perfection:** Celebrate small wins and recognize how far you've come.

  - **Example:** Lisa, an AuDHD student, would spend hours trying to make her essays absolutely perfect, often missing deadlines due to her perfectionism. She started practicing **self-compassion**, reminding herself, "My best is enough. It's okay if this isn't perfect; it just needs to be good enough." She also set a timer and stopped working on an assignment when the timer went off, forcing herself to accept "good enough." This dramatically reduced her stress and improved her ability to submit work on time.

Holistic self-care isn't about adding more items to your to-do list. It's about fundamentally shifting your approach to yourself and your needs. It's about recognizing that nurturing your body, mind, and spirit is not an indulgence, but a vital part of living a full and joyful life with AuDHD. By integrating these strategies, you equip yourself to prevent burnout and consistently cultivate genuine moments of joy.

Key Takeaways

- **Holistic self-care** is not a luxury but an indispensable strategy for managing AuDHD and preventing burnout.

- Prioritize **sleep** (consistent schedule, calming routine, optimized environment), **nutrition** (whole foods, hydration, regular meals), and **regular exercise** (enjoyable activities, consistency over intensity) as foundational elements.

- Establish **healthy boundaries** with yourself and others to protect your energy and prevent overwhelm, clearly communicating your limits.

- Engage in **personal interests and creative outlets** as powerful tools for emotional regulation, fostering joy, and harnessing **hyperfocus**.

- Practice **self-compassion** and let go of **perfectionistic tendencies**, treating yourself with kindness and accepting that "good enough" is often sufficient.

A Final Thought

Navigating life with AuDHD is a journey that asks for understanding, patience, and a willingness to see the world a bit differently. As you gather these tools for communication, support, emotional regulation, and self-care, remember this: your unique wiring is not something to be fixed, but something to be understood, celebrated, and nurtured. You have incredible strengths and a distinct way of experiencing joy. By embracing these practical strategies, you are not just coping; you are building a life designed by you, for you, full of genuine connection, purpose, and lasting well-being.

Chapter 11: Navigating Diagnosis & Professional Support

Understanding that you might have AuDHD, or even just wondering if you do, can be a moment of clarity and, sometimes, a bit overwhelming. It's like finding a new map to a place you've always lived but never quite understood. This map can help you see why certain roads felt bumpy, why some paths were easier, and why you sometimes felt lost. Getting an official diagnosis can be a significant step on this path, opening doors to understanding and support you might not have known existed. This part of our discussion will help you navigate that journey, from finding the right professionals to exploring the various ways they can help you build a life that truly works for you.

The journey to an AuDHD diagnosis as an adult can be a bit of a winding road. For many years, autism and ADHD were often seen as separate conditions, and adult diagnoses were not as common as they are today. This means that you might have spent years feeling "different" or "wrong" without a clear explanation. Getting a formal assessment can provide immense validation—a sense of relief that there's a reason for your experiences, and that you're not alone. It's about putting a name to what you've always felt and then finding the right support to help you thrive.

Finding Qualified Professionals for Assessment

The first step in getting a diagnosis is finding the right people to help you. This can be tricky, as not all mental health professionals are equipped to assess for both autism and ADHD in adults, especially when they co-occur. You need someone who truly understands **neurodiversity** and has experience with the subtle ways AuDHD can present in adults, which often differs from childhood presentations.

Here's a guide to finding a qualified professional:

1. **Look for Specialists in Adult Neurodevelopmental Conditions:** Do not settle for a general practitioner who might not have the specialized training. Seek out psychologists, psychiatrists, or neuropsychologists who specifically mention expertise in **adult autism (ASD)** and **Adult ADHD**. Even better if they mention experience with co-occurring conditions.

2. **Ask About Their Approach to AuDHD:** When you first contact a potential professional, ask direct questions:

   o "Do you assess for both autism and ADHD in adults?"

   o "Are you familiar with the concept of AuDHD or co-occurring autism and ADHD?"

   o "What is your approach to assessing individuals who might have both?"

   o "Are you neurodiversity-affirming?" (This means they see neurodiversity as a natural variation, not just a disorder to be "cured.")

3. **Consider Neuropsychological Evaluations:** These are often the most thorough assessments. A neuropsychologist will use a combination of interviews, questionnaires, and cognitive tests to get a full picture of your cognitive strengths and challenges, and how they relate to diagnostic criteria for both autism and ADHD.

4. **Seek Recommendations:**

   o **Online Neurodiversity Communities:** Ask for recommendations in online forums or social media groups dedicated to AuDHD or adult autism/ADHD. Other neurodivergent people often have excellent first-hand experience with practitioners.

   o **Disability Services Offices:** If you are a student or connected to a university, their disability services office might have a list of recommended evaluators.

   o **Neurodiversity-Affirming Organizations:** Look for local or national organizations that support neurodivergent individuals; they often provide directories or referral services.

5. **Be Prepared for a Process:** Getting an adult diagnosis can take time. It often involves multiple sessions, gathering historical information (sometimes from family members), and a detailed report. Be patient with the process.

For example, Sarah, a 35-year-old artist, always felt a bit "off" but couldn't place it. After reading about AuDHD online, she suspected it might be her. She first tried a general therapist who dismissed her concerns. Undeterred, Sarah then searched for "adult autism assessment" and "adult ADHD diagnosis" in her area, specifically looking for practitioners with "neurodiversity-affirming" in their descriptions. She found a clinical psychologist who specialized in adult neurodevelopmental conditions. During their initial call, Sarah asked specific questions about AuDHD. The psychologist's answers showed a genuine understanding, and Sarah felt comfortable moving forward with the assessment, which ultimately provided the clarity she sought.

Therapeutic Approaches and Medication Considerations

Once you have a diagnosis, or even if you're just exploring ways to manage AuDHD traits, several therapeutic approaches can be incredibly helpful. These therapies are not about changing who you are but about providing you with tools to navigate the world more effectively and reduce distress.

1. **Cognitive Behavioral Therapy (CBT):**

    o **What it is:** CBT helps you identify and challenge unhelpful thinking patterns and behaviors. It's often structured and goal-oriented.

    o **How it helps AuDHD:**

        ▪ **Managing negative self-talk:** For AuDHD individuals who have internalized decades of criticism, CBT can help reframe self-defeating thoughts.

        ▪ **Anxiety and depression:** It can be very effective for managing anxiety (common with autism) and depression (often linked to the executive dysfunction and overwhelm of ADHD).

        ▪ **Developing coping strategies:** It provides concrete strategies for

90

managing overwhelming situations or strong emotions.

- o **Example:** David (from a previous example) used CBT to address his intense frustration when plans changed unexpectedly. His therapist helped him identify the thought, "Changes are always bad and mean things will fall apart." They then worked on reframing it to, "Changes can be challenging, but I have coping tools, and I can adapt." This shifted his emotional response.

2. **Dialectical Behavior Therapy (DBT):**

- o **What it is:** DBT is a type of CBT that places a strong emphasis on emotional regulation, distress tolerance, interpersonal effectiveness, and mindfulness.

- o **How it helps AuDHD:**

    - **Emotional dysregulation:** Its focus on managing intense emotions (like those experienced during meltdowns) is incredibly helpful.

    - **Distress tolerance:** Teaches skills to get through crisis situations without making things worse.

    - **Interpersonal skills:** Helps with navigating relationships and communicating needs effectively.

- **Mindfulness:** Grounding techniques and present-moment awareness are central to DBT.

- Example: Emily, who experienced meltdowns, found DBT skills training very useful. She learned to use "TIPP" skills (Temperature, Intense exercise, Paced breathing, Paired muscle relaxation) to manage moments of extreme emotional arousal, giving her concrete actions to take when overwhelmed.

3. **Occupational Therapy (OT):**

   - **What it is:** OT focuses on helping you participate in the daily activities (occupations) that are important to you. It often involves sensory integration, executive function coaching, and practical strategies for daily living.

   - **How it helps AuDHD:**

     - **Sensory regulation:** An OT can help you understand your sensory profile and develop strategies (e.g., sensory diets, environmental modifications) to manage sensory input at home, work, or in public.

     - **Executive function support:** They can provide practical tools for organization, planning, time management, and task initiation.

- **Activities of daily living:** Help with routines around hygiene, meal prep, managing finances, etc.

- **Example:** Leo, who struggled with maintaining a consistent routine, worked with an OT. The OT helped him set up a visual schedule for his mornings, suggested noise-canceling headphones for his study time, and even advised on organizing his kitchen to make meal prep less overwhelming.

4. **Social Skills Training:**

   - **What it is:** This therapy focuses on teaching explicit social rules, conversational dynamics, and interpretation of social cues.

   - **How it helps AuDHD:** While the "Double Empathy Problem" [1] reminds us that social struggles are mutual, learning explicit social skills can help AuDHD individuals navigate neurotypical environments with less anxiety and more confidence. This is about acquiring tools, not changing who you are.

   - **Example:** Maria joined a social skills group where she learned about conversational turn-taking, asking open-ended questions, and understanding nuances in tone of voice. This helped her feel less anxious in professional networking situations.

5. **Medication Considerations:**

- For the ADHD aspects of AuDHD, **medication** (stimulants or non-stimulants) can be very effective in managing symptoms like inattention, impulsivity, and hyperactivity. It can help regulate dopamine and norepinephrine in the brain, improving focus and executive function.

- **Important Considerations:**

  - **Consult a psychiatrist:** Medication should always be prescribed and monitored by a qualified psychiatrist.

  - **Potential interactions:** Be aware that medication for ADHD can sometimes heighten sensory sensitivities or anxiety for autistic individuals, so a cautious approach and close monitoring are essential.

  - **Not a cure:** Medication helps manage symptoms, but it's not a standalone solution. It works best in conjunction with therapy and lifestyle strategies.

- **Example:** Mark, after his diagnosis, started on a low dose of ADHD medication. He found it significantly improved his focus at work and reduced his internal restlessness. However, he noticed it also made him more sensitive to bright lights, so he adjusted his office lighting and continued to use his noise-canceling headphones. His psychiatrist worked closely with him to find the right balance.

94

The AuDHD Coach: Practical, Individualized Support

Beyond traditional therapy, an **AuDHD coach** (or neurodiversity-affirming coach) can provide highly practical, individualized support. These coaches often have lived experience with neurodiversity themselves or are deeply trained in neurodivergent-affirming practices. They focus on helping you implement strategies in your daily life, achieve goals, and build executive function skills.

- **What a coach does:**
  - Helps you **set realistic goals** that align with your neurotype.
  - Provides **accountability** and structure.
  - Offers **practical strategies** for organization, time management, task initiation, and managing overwhelm.
  - Helps you **identify and leverage your strengths**.
  - Acts as a **sounding board** for challenges and triumphs.
  - Focuses on **current and future goals**, rather than past traumas (which is more the domain of therapy).

- **How it helps AuDHD:** A good AuDHD coach understands the unique interplay of autistic and ADHD traits. They can help you create systems that work *with* your brain, not against it. They understand the nuances of **hyperfocus**, sensory needs, and communication differences.

- **Finding a coach:** Look for coaches who specialize in neurodiversity, especially AuDHD. Ask about their training, their approach, and if they offer a free introductory call to see if it's a good fit. Certification from reputable coaching bodies is a plus.

For instance, Maria (from previous examples), while benefiting from her DBT skills, found herself still struggling with procrastination and organizing her creative projects. She hired an AuDHD coach. Her coach helped her break down her larger art projects into smaller steps, set up a simple visual task board, and taught her how to use "body doubling" to start difficult tasks. The coach didn't just tell her what to do; they worked with Maria to create systems that actually fit *her* brain, leading to increased productivity and less self-criticism.

Accessing professional support—whether it's through a formal diagnosis, therapy, medication, or coaching—is a proactive step toward creating a life where you not only manage your AuDHD but truly flourish because of it. It's about building a team around you that understands and empowers your unique way of being.

Key Takeaways

- Finding qualified professionals for **AuDHD assessment** involves seeking specialists in adult neurodevelopmental conditions, asking about their neurodiversity-affirming approach, considering neuropsychological evaluations, and seeking recommendations.

- **Therapeutic approaches** like CBT (for thought patterns, anxiety), DBT (for emotional regulation, distress tolerance), OT (for sensory and executive function support), and social skills training (for communication tools) offer practical strategies.

- **Medication** can help manage ADHD symptoms, but consultation with a psychiatrist is essential, with careful monitoring for autistic sensitivities.

- An **AuDHD coach** provides practical, individualized support, helping with goal setting, accountability, skill-building, and leveraging strengths.

Chapter 12: Living an AuDHD-Affirming Life

Your Future, Your Way

You have learned about your AuDHD, understood some of its unique workings, gathered tools for daily living, and explored avenues for professional support. What now? This final part of our discussion is about bringing all those pieces together. It's about recognizing that having AuDHD isn't a problem to be solved, but a unique way of being human that can be embraced and celebrated. It's about building a future that truly fits *you*, rather than trying to fit yourself into a mold that was never designed for your beautiful, complex brain. This means learning to advocate for yourself and planning for a life that supports your well-being and allows you to find sustained joy and fulfillment.

Self-Advocacy: Articulating Your Needs and Preferences

Self-advocacy is your superpower. It's the ability to speak up for yourself, to articulate your needs, preferences, and boundaries in a clear and respectful way. For AuDHD individuals, who may have been misunderstood or had their needs dismissed for years, learning to self-advocate is a liberating skill. It puts you in the driver's seat of your own life.

Self-advocacy applies to every area of your life:

- **In Relationships:** "I need 30 minutes of quiet time after work before we talk about anything important." or "I process information better if you tell me directly what you need, rather than hinting."

- **At Work:** "To help me focus, I need to use my noise-canceling headphones during deep work periods." or "Could I get instructions for this project in writing, please?"

- **In Public Spaces:** "Could we sit at a table away from the speakers? I'm sensitive to loud noises." or "I need to leave this event now; I'm feeling overwhelmed."

- **With Healthcare Providers:** "I need a doctor who understands neurodiversity. Can you tell me about your experience with AuDHD patients?" or "I prefer to have my appointments at the start of the day because my energy is higher then."

The Framework for Self-Advocacy:

1. **Know Yourself:** Understand your AuDHD traits, your strengths, your challenges, your sensory sensitivities, and your energy limits. What helps you thrive? What depletes you?

2. **Know Your Needs:** Based on self-knowledge, identify specific needs related to environments, communication, routines, and support.

3. **Communicate Clearly:**

   - **Be Direct:** Avoid vague language.

   - **Use "I" Statements:** Focus on your experience ("I feel," "I need") rather than blaming ("You always...").

   - **Explain (Briefly):** Offer a concise explanation of *why* you have a certain need, if appropriate. This helps others understand. "I need quiet time because my brain processes sounds differently, and too much noise causes me to feel drained."

- ○ **Offer Solutions:** If possible, suggest practical ways to meet your need.

4. **Be Assertive, Not Aggressive:** State your needs calmly and confidently. You have a right to your needs.

5. **Accept Not Everyone Will Understand:** Some people may not respond positively. This reflects on them, not on the validity of your needs. Focus on those who *do* listen and support you.

For example, Mark (the man who started the electronics repair business) had a close friend, Chris, who often made spontaneous plans. Mark, with his AuDHD need for predictability, found this incredibly stressful. Mark decided to self-advocate: "Chris, I really value our friendship, but my brain works best with a bit more notice for plans. Could you please try to give me at least 24 hours' notice before we make plans? It helps me manage my energy and look forward to our time together, rather than feeling rushed and stressed." Chris, understanding Mark's needs, agreed, and their friendship grew stronger because of this clear communication.

Embracing Neurodiversity as a Strength

This is the heart of living an AuDHD-affirming life: viewing your neurodivergence not as a deficit, but as a **strength** and a **unique, valuable way of being human**. The world needs different kinds of minds to solve its problems, create beauty, and move forward. Your AuDHD brain comes with inherent advantages:

- **Originality:** You see connections and patterns others miss, leading to innovative ideas.

- **Depth of Interest:** Your capacity for **hyperfocus** allows you to become exceptionally knowledgeable and skilled in areas you care about.

- **Authenticity:** Many AuDHD individuals value honesty and directness, which can build truly meaningful connections.

- **Perseverance:** When genuinely engaged, your persistence can be unmatched.

- **Attention to Detail:** You might notice critical nuances that others overlook.

- **Justice-Oriented:** Your strong sense of fairness can drive positive change.

Embracing neurodiversity means letting go of the pressure to **mask** (hide your autistic and ADHD traits to fit in). Masking is incredibly exhausting and can lead to burnout, anxiety, and a loss of self. While some masking may be necessary in certain situations, the goal is to reduce it wherever possible and to find spaces where you can be your authentic self.

Celebrate your differences! You don't need to be "fixed." You need understanding, support, and environments that accommodate your natural way of being.

Long-Term Planning for Well-being and Fulfillment

Living an AuDHD-affirming life isn't just about coping day-to-day; it's about setting yourself up for long-term well-being and fulfillment. This involves integrating all the strategies we've discussed throughout this book into a cohesive framework for your life.

1. **Regularly Review Your Self-Care Plan:** Your needs may change over time. What worked last year might not work today. Regularly assess your sleep, nutrition, exercise, and sensory needs. Are you getting enough quiet time? Are your special interests still engaging you? Adjust as needed.

2. **Build a Neurodiversity-Affirming Environment:** Actively shape your home, work, and social environments to support your AuDHD. This might mean:

   o **Home:** Creating sensory-friendly spaces, organizing systems that work for you (even if unconventional), and having quiet zones.

   o **Work:** Continuing to advocate for accommodations, seeking roles that align with your strengths, or exploring self-employment if traditional work is too draining.

   o **Social:** Cultivating relationships with people who genuinely understand and accept you, and limiting time with those who don't.

3. **Continuously Develop Your Coping Tools:** Keep practicing mindfulness, deep breathing, and grounding techniques. Explore new ones. The more tools you have in your emotional regulation toolkit, the better equipped you'll be for life's challenges.

4. **Embrace Learning and Growth:** See learning about yourself, your AuDHD, and the world as an ongoing adventure. Stay curious, engage with your special interests, and keep building new skills.

5. **Plan for "Recharge" Periods:** Regularly schedule downtime, sensory breaks, and focused engagement with your special interests. These are not luxuries; they are essential for preventing burnout and maintaining mental health. Think of them as non-negotiable appointments with yourself.

6. **Seek Joy Intentionally:** Don't wait for joy to find you. Actively seek out activities, connections, and experiences that bring you genuine happiness and a sense of purpose. This might be pursuing a passion project, spending time in nature, connecting with neurokin, or engaging in creative expression.

For example, Lisa, after years of struggling with burnout in her demanding career, realized she needed a drastic change to truly live an AuDHD-affirming life. She identified that her need for autonomy and deep work without interruptions was not being met. She worked with her AuDHD coach to plan a transition from her corporate job to freelancing in her field, allowing her to set her own hours, choose projects that aligned with her interests, and work from a quiet home office. This long-term planning, integrating her understanding of her AuDHD, enabled her to create a sustainable and fulfilling career that honored her unique operating system.

Additional Resources for Your Journey

This journey of understanding and living an AuDHD-affirming life is ongoing. Here are some resources to help you continue your learning and connect with others:

- **Recommended Books:**
    - *Unmasking Autism: Discovering the New Faces of Neurodiversity* by Devon Price [2]
    - *Divergent Mind: Thriving in a World That Wasn't Designed For You* by Jenara Nerenberg [3]
    - *The ADHD Effect on Marriage* by Melissa Orlov (While focused on marriage, it offers valuable insights into ADHD traits in relationships) [4]
    - *Neurotribes: The Legacy of Autism and How to Think Smarter About People Who Think Differently* by Steve Silberman [5]

- **Online Communities:**
    - **Reddit:** Subreddits like r/AuDHD, r/autism, r/ADHD offer spaces for connection and shared experiences.
    - **Facebook Groups:** Search for "AuDHD adult support" or "neurodiversity affirmation" groups.
    - **Discord Servers:** Many neurodivergent communities host Discord servers for real-time chat and support.

- **Reputable Organizations:**

- o **Autistic Self Advocacy Network (ASAN):** A non-profit organization run by and for autistic people, focusing on advocacy and policy. [6]

- o **CHADD (Children and Adults with Attention-Deficit/Hyperactivity Disorder):** Provides education, advocacy, and support for individuals with ADHD. [7]

- o **Neurodiversity Hub:** Offers resources for neurodivergent individuals in education and employment. [8]

Key Takeaways

- **Self-advocacy** is a vital skill for AuDHD individuals across all areas of life, involving knowing your needs, communicating them clearly using "I" statements, and offering solutions.

- **Embracing neurodiversity as a strength** means recognizing your unique advantages (originality, depth of interest, authenticity) and reducing masking to live authentically.

- **Long-term planning** for well-being includes regularly reviewing self-care, building neurodiversity-affirming environments, continuously developing coping tools, embracing learning, scheduling recharge periods, and intentionally seeking joy.

- Further **resources** like recommended books, online communities, and reputable organizations can support your ongoing journey of understanding and thriving.

A Parting Thought

Living a fulfilling life with AuDHD is not about erasing your traits or trying to be someone you're not. It's about a fundamental shift in perspective—seeing your unique brain wiring as a source of strength, creativity, and a distinctive way of moving through the world. By gathering tools, building supportive networks, and boldly advocating for your needs, you can design a life that truly embraces who you are, allowing your most authentic self to shine brightly. Your future is yours to shape, with all its wonderful neurodivergent brilliance.

References

1. American Psychiatric Association. (2013). *Diagnostic and Statistical Manual of Mental Disorders* (5th ed.). Arlington, VA: American Psychiatric Publishing.

2. Price, D. (2022). *Unmasking Autism: Discovering the New Faces of Neurodiversity*. Penguin Random House.

3. McCabe, J. (2023). *How to ADHD: An Insider's Guide to Working with Your Brain (Not Against It)*. Penguin Life.

4. Hopkins, L. (2022). *Understanding AuDHD: A comprehensive guide*. Independently Published.

5. Sadiq, K. (2024). *Explaining AuDHD: The expert-led guide to Autism and ADHD Co-concurrence*. Jessica Kingsley Publishers.

6. Maskell, L. (2024). *AuDHD: Blooming Differently*. Welbeck Balance.

7. Havas PR. (2023, April 19). *Havas PR Announces Neurodiversity Report Showing Neurodivergent Consumers Expect Brands to Engage with Them and Meet Their Needs*. PR Newswire.

8. Routledge. (n.d.). *Neurodiversity in the Workplace*. Retrieved from [Routledge Academic Publishers website on neurodiversity in the workplace - actual URL not available to Browse tool during research].

9. Brown, T. E. (2014). *Smart but stuck: Emotions in teens and adults with ADHD*. Jossey-Bass.

10. Dunn, W. (1997). The impact of sensory processing abilities on the daily lives of young children and their families: A conceptual model. *Infants & Young Children*, 9(4), 23-35.

11. Dawson, G., & Osterling, J. (1997). Early recognition of autism: A developmental perspective. *Developmental Psychopathology*, 9(3), 439-450.

12. Barkley, R. A. (2015). *Attention-deficit hyperactivity disorder: A handbook for diagnosis and treatment* (4th ed.). Guilford Press.

13. Miller, L. J., & Lane, S. J. (2000). Toward a consensus of sensory modulation disorder. *Sensory Integration Special Interest Section Quarterly*, 23(2), 1-4.

14. Russel, A., et al. (2020). The intersection of ADHD and autism: A review of the literature. *Journal of Autism and Developmental Disorders*, 50(6), 2111-2125.

15. Milton, D. E. (2012). **"The 'double empathy problem': Ten years on."** *Autism*, 26(1), 12-14.

16. Price, D. (2022). **"Unmasking Autism: Discovering the New Faces of Neurodiversity."** *Penguin Random House*.

17. Nerenberg, J. (2020). **"Divergent Mind: Thriving in a World That Wasn't Designed For You."** *HarperOne*.

18. Orlov, M. (2010). **"The ADHD Effect on Marriage: Understand and Rebuild Your Relationship in Six Steps."** *Specialty Press, Inc.*

19. Silberman, S. (2015). **"NeuroTribes: The Legacy of Autism and How to Think Smarter About People Who Think Differently."** *Avery*.

20. Autistic Self Advocacy Network (ASAN). **"About ASAN."** Available at: https://autisticadvocacy.org/about-asan/

21. CHADD (Children and Adults with Attention-Deficit/Hyperactivity Disorder). **"About CHADD."** Available at: https://chadd.org/about/

22. Neurodiversity Hub. **"About Us."** Available at: https://neurodiversityhub.org/about-us/